Calculations and Pharmaceutics in Practice

*This book is dedicated to the memory of Roy Edward Watson
(17.12.1935 – 2.2.2019).*

As all teachers are, he was tremendously proud of his pupils. When he died, more than thirty years after he had retired, many former pupils shared their memories of him with us. As educators, we should all hope to be remembered in this way.

He was also proud of his wife, children and grandson. He was tickled pink to get his hands on the 5th edition of Pharmaceutical Practice *with his daughter's name on the front of it.*

Thank you Dad; one of the best teachers I have ever had.

'No man dies unless he is forgotten.'

Calculations and Pharmaceutics in Practice

Edited by

Jennie Watson
BSc, PG ClinDip, PGCert (LTHE), FFRPS, MRPharmS, FHEA

Boots Teacher/Practitioner, School of Pharmacy and Biomedical Sciences,
University of Central Lancashire, Preston, UK

Louise Cogan
BSc (Hons), PG Dip, PGCert (LTHE), PG Cert (Research and Evaluation)
MRPharmS, FHEA

Senior Lecturer, School of Pharmacy and Biomedical Sciences,
University of Central Lancashire, Preston, UK

For additional online content visit StudentConsult.com

ELSEVIER   Edinburgh   London   New York   Oxford   Philadelphia   St Louis   Sydney   2020

First edition 2020

Notices

Practitioners and researchers must always rely on their own experience and knowledge in evaluating and using any information, methods, compounds or experiments described herein. Because of rapid advances in the medical sciences, in particular, independent verification of diagnoses and drug dosages should be made. To the fullest extent of the law, no responsibility is assumed by Elsevier, authors, editors or contribu-tors for any injury and/or damage to persons or property as a matter of products liability, negligence or otherwise, or from any use or operation of any methods, products, instructions, or ideas contained in the material herein.

ISBN: 978-0-7020-7439-4

Content Strategist: Pauline Graham
Content Development Specialist: Fiona Conn
Project Manager: Julie Taylor
Design: Brian Salisbury
Marketing Manager: Deborah Watkins

Printed in Poland

Last digit is the print number: 9 8 7 6 5 4 3 2 1

Working together to grow libraries in developing countries

www.elsevier.com • www.bookaid.org

Contents

Preface

Whilst the majority of pharmacists still work in the traditional employment area of hospital and community pharmacy, these roles continue to evolve and more pharmacists are moving to work in new and emerging roles, including working in GP practices, care settings and hospital emergency departments. Some of these new roles include prescribing and many are related to the increasing focus on medicines optimization.

We recognize, however, that pharmacists in the UK and elsewhere in the world are still involved in the production of medicines either within the pharmaceutical industry or through smaller scale compounding in their pharmacies. This has led to this book, which contains the chapters from *Pharmacy Practice* sixth edition (Elsevier 2020) that relate to pharmaceutical preparation and calculations.

Our contributors have been chosen for their expertise and experience. They include practising pharmacists, academics and some who work between practice and academia.

For readers who require greater detail on the scientific principles that underpin the design and manufacture of dosage forms and medicines, we would recommend *Aulton's Pharmaceutics: The Design and Manufacture of Medicines,* fifth edition (Churchill Livingstone 2017), edited by M.E. Aulton and K. Taylor. Readers should realize that information cannot be compartmentalized. It is detrimental to patients to ignore any aspect of the total knowledge base and so we would encourage you to read around any specialist area to ensure optimum patient care.

JW, LSC

Acknowledgements

The editors would like to take this opportunity to thank the many people who have helped to make this book possible. Since publication of the fifth edition of the parent book, *Pharmacy Practice*, both Dr Judith A. Rees and Ian Smith have decided to 'retire' as editors. Judy and Ian were very experienced authors and editors and had worked on two editions of this book. I (JW) felt that they would be hard to replace and I know all three of us had doubts about the wisdom of two thirds of the editorial team leaving at the same time. Fortunately, I was able to find a willing and able replacement in Louise Cogan. We have worked well together and she has added new insights to the editorial process.

We are deeply grateful to all the authors for their willingness to contribute and for the time and effort they have spent researching their subjects and in preparing text. In particular, we would like to thank them for adhering to the timescales we gave them to complete their chapters – it must seem a long time from writing a chapter to seeing the book in print.

Our special thanks are due to our families. Without their continued encouragement, support and assistance, an undertaking like this would never reach completion. We apologise if on occasions, you have not received the attention you deserve.

Those companies, organizations and individuals who have given permission to use or modify their materials or who have helpfully answered queries or provided information to our authors are thanked. Without this type of cooperation, any textbook cannot hope to present a worthwhile overview.

Thanks are also expressed to the publishers, both Pauline Graham and Fiona Conn. Fiona in particular has had to deal with our queries, misunderstandings, etc., but has provided guidance, support and, on occasions, challenge with both great kindness and patience. We have also appreciated her quick response to questions through the publisher's electronic manuscript submission system – a wonderful invention.

Finally, we wish to thank you, our students both past and present. You cannot appreciate how much we learn from you and hope that some of this is reflected in this book.

JW, LSC

Contributors

Derek G. Chapman, BSc(Pharm), PhD
Retired Lecturer, Robert Gordon University, Aberdeen, UK

David Graham, BSc, MSc, MRPharmS
Radiopharmacy Team Leader, Radiopharmacy Department, Aberdeen Royal Infirmary, Aberdeen, UK

Lindsay Harper, BSc(Hons), DipClin
Principal Clinical Pharmacist, Pharmacy Department, Salford Royal NHS Foundation Trust, Salford, UK

Liz Lamerton, BSc(Hons) Pharmacy, DipClinPharm, PIP, FFRPS
Principal Clinical Pharmacist, Salford Royal NHS Foundation Trust, Salford, UK

Judith A. Rees, BPharm, MSc, PhD
Senior Lecturer, School of Pharmacy, Keele University, Keele, UK

R. Michael E. Richards, OBE, BPharm, PhD, DSc, DPharmSci(Honorary), DPharmPractice(Honorary)
Professor Emeritus, Pharmacy, Robert Gordon University, Aberdeen, UK; Professor of Pharmacy, Mahasarakham University, Maha Sarakham, Thailand

Peter M. Richards, BPharm (Hons)
Prescribing Adviser and Medicines Management Lead at Newark and Sherwood Clinical Commissioning Group, UK

Geoff Saunders, BPharm, MPhil
Pharmacy Specialist Education Lead Northwest, HEE, Manchester, UK

Ian Smith, BSc(Hons), MRPharmS, ClinDip, ILTM
Lecturer, School of Pharmacy, Keele University, Keele, UK

Jennie Watson, BSc, PG Clin Dip, PGCert(LTHE), MRPharmS
Boots Teacher Practitioner, School of Pharmacy and Biomedical Sciences, University of Central Lancashire, Preston, UK

Arthur J. Winfield, BPharm, PhD
Retired Senior Lecturer and Head of Pharmacy Practice, Robert Gordon University, Aberdeen, UK; Retired Chairman of Department of Pharmacy Practice, University of Kuwait, Kuwait

Chapter | 1 |

Using calculations in pharmacy practice

Jennie Watson

STUDY POINTS

- To understand the significance of units
- To consider types of calculations and where they are used in practice

Introduction

In pharmacy we are, on occasions, required to carry out calculations. How many calculations you may need to do on a daily or weekly basis will vary depending on the role you have. Understanding how to carry out calculations accurately is very important in terms of patient safety and so it is important to understand when you may need to do a calculation and how to carry it out.

Why are units important?

Most units of measurement used in health care in most countries are metric measurements. Some measurements, particularly weight and height, may be given in imperial measurements, especially when the patient provides the information. It is important that we know the units, as the changes between units in the metric system are by a factor of 1000, so if we get the unit wrong, we will have done significant harm to our patient with a substantial under or overdose.

Comparable sizes of units

In many calculations, you have a mixture of weights and volumes. To ensure that the calculation is correct, you need to use comparably sized units. This is usually grams and millilitres. It may help to remember which units to use by thinking about measuring and weighing water. If you were to pour 1 mL of water onto a scale pan, it would weigh about 1 g, so these are the comparable units as they are physically similar.

Converting between units and measurement systems

When using metric units, there is a factor of 1000 between each adjacent pair of units.

Weight
kg>g>mg>mcg
Volume
L>mL

When you change between units, the number changes by a factor of 1000, so this means if the unit gets smaller, the number gets bigger so:

2 kg = 2000 g = 2,000,000 mg = 2,000,000,000 mcg

Or if the unit gets bigger, the number gets smaller:

8 mcg = 0.008 mg = 0.000008 g = 0.00000008 kg

If we need to change between systems of units, we need to find the conversion factor. An example is:

1 inch = 2.54 cm, so if we know a height in inches, we can convert it to cm by multiplying the number by 2.54.

Rounding

Rounding is needed on occasions to give practical quantities for both administration and supply. It is important, however, not round too early in a calculation. If you are

1

using a calculator, you should really continue to use all the decimal places to the end of the calculation and then round.

If your answer is less than 0.5 then round down to the nearest whole number.

If your answer is 0.5 or more then round up to the nearest whole number.

The main exception to this rule is in chemotherapy doses. Chemotherapy doses are often written as a maximum dose in mg/kg of body weight. If the answer is then rounded up, then the patient will be above this maximum dose. Since chemotherapy is in its nature highly toxic, this will cause harm.

Sense checking your answer

It is always important to check your answers. You may be able to do this by getting a colleague to also work out the calculation, but if you do not have anyone with you who can do this, then you need an alternative way to check. This may be carrying out another task before returning to the calculation and doing it again, possibly using a different method. You may also be able to 'sense check' your answer. This is where you consider whether your answer seems reasonable. Whilst this will be no total guarantee of success, you should at least ensure you are not a factor of 1000 out – see 'Why are units important?'.

Examples of how to 'sense check' include:
- If we have diluted a product, the final amount must be more than we started with
- Doses must feel sensible, if we have calculated the dose as 57.65 mL of an oral medicine for a baby, this does not 'feel' right for two reasons, firstly this is a large amount of over 11 × 5 mL spoonfuls which is not practical to administer to a baby, secondly, we cannot ask a parent to measure a volume at home to two decimal places
- We have decided that the right answer is dissolve 900 g of solid in 200 mL of liquid. This will not be physically possible, think about supersaturated solutions.

How to write strengths

Strengths are written in a variety of forms:
1. As quantity in quantity, such as 0.5 g in 100 mL. This is a physical recognition of how much of something is in a larger quantity
2. As parts. There are two ways to describe parts:
   1 part: 4 parts or 1 part to 4 parts
   here we have 5 parts in total, so our one part is 1/5 or 20%
   1 part in 4 parts
   here we have 4 parts in total, so our one part is 1/4 or 25%

3. As a percentage. When we use percentages, we are always talking about a number of something in 100.

Again, we need to remember to use comparable sized units if the product is made from a mixture of weights and volumes.

We also need to remember the following nomenclature:
W/W is where the active ingredient is measured as a weight and so is the total quantity
W/V is where the active ingredient is measured as a weight and the total quantity is measured as a volume
V/W is where the active ingredient is measured as a volume and the total quantity is measured as a weight
V/V is where the active ingredient is measured as a volume and so it the total quantity.

Doses and dosing

Drugs are usually prescribed in doses of milligrams or millilitres, it does not matter however, which units you are using as long as they are consistent. Some large molecules (such as insulin and some other hormones) are prescribed in units.

Patient specifics

Sometimes the dose is described in terms of one of the patient's body measurements:
- mg/kg – this is where the second number is the weight of the patient (often used in children)
- mg/m^2 – this is where the second number is the body surface area of the patient (most likely in children, the elderly or for chemotherapy)
- Ideal body weight. This is used for drugs that are totally or almost totally water-soluble and so the volume of distribution for the drug is not increased in a fatter patient. A common example of a drug with this pattern of distribution is gentamycin.

How much should be given?

It is important that the patient receives the correct amount of medicine. Too little and they will be inconvenienced and may also stop treatment prematurely. Too much and the patient may take a longer course of treatment than intended.

These calculations are often straightforward and rely on you understanding the relevant dose abbreviations and how to multiply, usually by 28.

An example would be a prescription that states:

1 tds for 28 days

This means one tablet three times a day for 28 days, so the calculation is

$$3 \times 28 = 84$$

Some doses are reducing and so the calculation is a little more complicated and you may need to write out the number of tablets each day to work out the quantity to supply.

An example would a prescription that states:

Prednisolone 30 mg daily for 10 days and then reduce by 5 mg every third day until at 0 mg. How many tablets do you need?

The other point that would need to be considered in this case is the strength of tablets available – 5 mg or 1 mg. It would not be practical for a patient to take 30 × 1mg tablets a day, so would be supplied with 5-mg tablets with a starting dose of six tablets on day 1.

Total to supply:

Days 1 – 10, six per day for 10 days = 60 tablets
Days 11 – 13, five per day for 3 days = 15 tablets
Days 14 – 16, four per day for 3 days = 12 tablets
Days 17 – 19, three per day for 3 days = 9 tablets
Days 20 – 22, two per day for 3 days = 6 tablets
Days 23 – 25, one per day for 3 days = 3 tablets
Total = 60 + 15 + 12 + 9 + 6 + 3 = 105 tablets

Calculations involving dilutions

When diluting a product, you will always have more of the final product than you started with. Some calculations involving dilutions will require multiple dilutions to reach the final product (see Ch. 10).

Dilutions can be used for liquid products (e.g. solutions or suspensions) or for solid products (e.g. creams, powders).

Simple dilutions

These are where only one dilution is needed to move from the initial product to the final product. Depending on the product, the strengths will be described as a percentage, a unit strength (e.g. x mg/5 mL) or in parts.

There are two main ways to calculate dilutions:

1. Stepwise: where you keep calculate the changes at each step of the calculation. For example:
   What volume of a 40% w/v solution needs to be used to produce 500 mL of a 5% w/v solution?
   5% is 5 g in 100 mL
   Or 25 g in 500 mL (remember to always do the same multiplication or division to each side of the formula)
   Therefore we need 25 g of the active ingredient and we need to get this from our 40% stock solution
   40% is 40 g in 100 mL or

10 g in 25 mL or
5 g in 12.5 mL
If we want 25 g we need to add together
10 g in 25 mL +
10 g in 25 mL +
5 g in 12.5 mL = 62.5 mL
25 g in 62.5 mL

2. Using a quadratic equation: (C1V1 = C2V2, where C1 is the concentration of the initial product, V1 is the volume of the initial product, C2 is the concentration of the final product and V2 is the volume of the final product. Providing you keep the units and strength format the same, if you know three of the values, you can calculate the missing value).

Complex dilutions

In these calculations, the simple dilution described earlier is repeated more than once.

These would be used in one of the following situations:

1. Where the amount of the product needed is too small to measure in one step (see Ch. 10)
2. Where the last stage of the dilution is carried out by the patient, either because the final product is unstable and so has a limited shelf life from preparation or because the final product would be an impractically large volume.

The following is a fairly typical multiple dilution question

A 74-year-old woman needs to clean a foot ulcer with potassium permanganate solution. How much potassium permanganate would be required to produce 200 mL of a solution so that when 5 mL of the solution is diluted to 1 litre it gives a strength of 1 in 5000?

To carry out these calculations, you always work backwards from the final product. For the aforementioned question, this would mean:

Final product contains 1 in 5000, i.e. 1g in 5000 mL
If we have 1 litre of this, the amount of potassium permanganate is 1/5 of 1 g, i.e. 0.2 g
We know that this 0.2 g is also in 5 mL of our original solution as the active ingredient in the final product can only have come from this amount of the original solution.
Therefore the original product we need to make is at a strength of
0.2 g in 5 mL
If we need 200 mL of this original solution, we know it must contain
0.2 g in 5 mL
2 g in 50 mL
8 g in 200 mL
So the answer is 8 g.

Infusion rates and volumes

How and why infusions are administered

Infusions are when volumes of liquid medicines are administered over a period of time because of the volume needed (perhaps electrolytes) or because the patient needs a continuous amount of the drug or fluid (for example pain relief). Infusions are also of use if the patient is unable to swallow, for example they are unconscious.

There are two main types of device used to administer infusions:

1. An infusion giving set or pump. These infuse liquid into a vein by gravity or pumped electrically at a certain rate. The infusion rate is measured in volume (mL or drips) in a period of time (minutes or hours). These are usually used for fluids, blood products or drugs such as antibiotics.
2. A syringe driver. These infuse liquid into a vein by electrically depressing a syringe as a certain rate. The infusion rate is measured in distance (mm or cm) that the syringe plunger moves in a period of time (minutes or hours). These are usually used for controlled drug delivery as the syringe itself can be locked into a secure container attached to the wall.

Infusion rates

Infusion rates describe how much of the drug/product is administered over a period of time

Simple volume/minute

One litre of saline solution is to be given to a patient over a 6-hour period. If each mL contains 20 drops, how many drops per minute should be administered?

The answer needs to be in minutes, so 6 hours = 360 minutes
If there are 20 drops in 1 mL then
There are 20 × 1000 in 1000 mL or 20,000
We are therefore administering 20,000 drops in 360 minutes or
20,000/360 drops in 1 minute
This gives 56 (55.5 but you cannot give half a drop) drops in 1 minute, so
The infusion rate is 56 drops/min.

Adding drugs to infusion bags

In these calculations, a drug is added to a full infusion bag. To do this practically, the same volume would need first to be removed using an aseptic technique to allow enough space in the bag for the drug to be added. Calculation questions of this type look complicated but provided they are considered in relation to practice, rather than purely mathematical, they are logical to complete.

A dopamine infusion is to be started for a child who weighs 10 kg. The doctor would like to administer 5 mcg/kg/min but would like to administer the fluids at 10 mL/h. You have 250-mL bags of glucose 5% and pre-filled syringes of dopamine 200 mg/5 mL.

How many mL of the dopamine solution would need to be added to the 250-mL bag of glucose 5% in order to infuse the dopamine at the requested dose and fluid rate? (Give your answer to 3 decimal places).

The first thing is not to panic but to think about what you are actually being asked to do in practice rather than just as a theoretical calculation.
How much drug do you need to give?
5 mcg/kg/min for a 10-kg child = 50 mcg/min
The other piece of information we have that includes time is in mL/h, so we need to covert the amount of time into hours:
50 mcg/min is (50 × 60) mcg/h or 3000 mcg/h or 3 mg/h
If our flow rate is 10 mL/h then we will be giving 3 mg of drug in every 10 mL, so the final strength in the infusion bag must be 3 mg/10 mL
If our infusion bag is 250 mL in total, we can calculate the total amount of drug in the bag:
3 mg in 10 mL
(3 × 25) mg in 250 mL
Or 75 mg in 250 mL
We then need to work out how much of the pre-filled dopamine syringe we need to provide 75 mg
Dopamine is 200 mg/5 mL or 40 mg/mL
If we need 75 mg, we need 75 ÷ 40 = 1.875 mL (and sense checking this we know it must be just less than 2 mL)
Therefore we will remove 1.875 mL of glucose from the infusion bag and replace with 1.875 mL of dopamine.

Syringe drivers

These are big syringes, for example containing 300 mL of liquid. If the syringe plunger was 20-cm long, then every time the plunger moves by 1 cm it administers one 20th of the volume, i.e. 1.5 mL. They are used for controlled drugs as they can be physically locked to a wall. If we know the strength of the solution, then we know how much drug is in a specific volume and therefore in distance travelled by the syringe plunger.

A patient is to receive 5 mg/h of morphine sulphate via a syringe driver. If the syringe driver contains 300 mL of morphine sulphate 2 mg/mL. The syringe length is 30 cm.

Calculate the flow rate in cm/h (give your answer to 2 decimal places).

To start with, calculate the total amount of drug in the syringe driver.

Strength is 2 mg/mL and total volume is 300 mL, therefore total amount of drug is 2 × 300 = 600 mg.

If the syringe length is 30 cm then for every cm the plunger moves, (600 ÷ 30 mg) 20 mg of drug will be administered.

So we know we need 5 mg/h and the strength of the solution is 20 mg/cm, so the flow rate will be:

5 ÷ 20 = 0.25 cm/h

Displacement values and volumes

Displacement volumes – solids dissolved in liquids

Displacement volumes relate to the amount of 'space' a solid occupies when it is dissolved in a liquid.

5 mL of liquid + 95 mL of liquid = 100 mL of liquids

5 g of solid + 95 mL of liquid = unknown volume which could be more or less than 100 mL

We know that the solid dissolves but we do not know how much additional space (above the 95 mL of liquid we already have) that it will take up.

However, the displacement volume of any solid in any liquid can be calculated after measurement and its units are mL/g.

The simplest way to think of this is to make up a bottle of antibiotic suspension from a powder.

Amoxicillin 125 mg/5 mL needs about 85 mL of water to make up 100 mL, so the amoxicillin 'fits into' 15 mL of the final 100 mL

Erythromycin 125 mg/5 mL needs about 80 mL of water to make up 100 mL, so the erythromycin 'fits into' 20 mL of the final 100 mL

Therefore erythromycin displaces more water than amoxicillin and will have a higher displacement value.

In practice, you would most commonly use this information for:

- Reconstituting antibiotic powders for children
- Reconstituting powders for injection such as diamorphine.

Displacement values – solids in solids

These values are very much dependent on density.

One gram of a heavy metal such as mercury will occupy much less volume than 1 g of a fluffy crystalline powder such as benzoic acid.

These values tend to matter when making something that needs to be a fixed size, such as a suppository where the mould volume is pre-determined.

Most displacement values relate to the amount of theobroma oil (a standard suppository base).

For example:

The displacement value of zinc oxide is 4.7. This means that 4.7 g of zinc oxide will displace (or occupy the space) of 1 g of theobroma oil, so zinc oxide is 4.7 times more dense than theobroma oil.

The displacement value of menthol is 0.7. This means that 0.7 g of menthol will displace 1 g of theobroma oil and so menthol is less dense than theobroma oil.

Calculations of kidney function

The kidney is involved in the excretion of most drugs or their metabolites. If the kidney does not work as well as expected (during illness or in the elderly), this can mean that the drug is not removed from the body as fast as expected and so can start to build up in the body. This means that doses may either have to be reduced or given less frequently.

Calculation of estimated creatinine clearance in a patient can be done using the Cockcroft and Gault formula, which is stated in the BNF.

$$\text{Estimated creatinine clearance in mL/min} = \frac{(140 - \text{age}) \times \text{Weight} \times \text{Constant}}{\text{Serum Creatinine}}$$

The age is in years

The weight should be the ideal body weight in kilograms

The constant = 1.23 for a man and 1.04 for a woman

The serum creatinine is micromol/L

Pharmacokinetics

Pharmacokinetic calculations are designed to try to optimize the dose of a drug for an individual patient to maximize its clinical effect whilst minimizing the risk of side-effects. The serum concentration that achieves these levels occurs within a range called the therapeutic window or index.

Most drugs have a wide therapeutic index and so standard doses tend to achieve serum concentrations within this range. Some drugs however, have what is described as a narrow therapeutic index and so a small change in dose, formulation or the body metabolism of the drug can alter the serum concentration from sub-therapeutic to toxic or vice versa very quickly. Examples of such drugs are phenytoin and gentamicin.

Bioavailability

This is the fraction of the drug that reaches the systemic circulation and can be affected by:

- Drugs that are metabolized in the stomach or liver tend to have low bioavailability
- Drugs that are subject to high first pass effects tend to have low bioavailability
- Drugs where different formulations or routes of administration release different amounts of drugs.

An example is the difference between digoxin tablets and elixir:

Drug and formulation	Approximate bioavailability
Digoxin tablets	0.7
Digoxin elixir	0.77

This means that you get about 10% more circulating digoxin from the same dose of elixir compared to tablets. Since this is a drug with a narrow therapeutic index, if the dose is not changed when the formulation is changed, then the patient could experience toxic side-effects.

$$\text{Oral dose} = \text{Amount systemically asborbed from standard formulation}$$

$$F \text{ (bioavailability)} \times S \text{ (salt fraction)}$$

Volume of distribution

How the drug is distributed around the body depends on how soluble it is between lipid and water. This distribution can take time and the time taken depends on the drug. This affects when the measurement is taken. An example is lithium, another drug with a narrow therapeutic index. It reaches its maximum dose 12 hours after administration. It is therefore taken at night so that the therapeutic drug monitoring can happen 12 hours later.

If a drug is almost entirely water-soluble (e.g. gentamycin), you will need to use the ideal body weight to calculate the dose. If you use the actual body weight, you will give the patient a higher dose than they need as the whole dose will only be distributed in the water compartment of the body and so the patient will receive an overdose.

$$\text{Volume of distribution } (V_d) =$$
$$\text{Amount of drug systemically absorbed}$$

$$\text{Serum concentration}$$

Elimination half-life

This is the time for the serum concentration of the drug to reduce by 50% ($T_{1/2}$).

Whilst the half-life can happen in non-linear way, most drugs follow a first order elimination and so if the amount of drug at time zero is 100%, the reduction in the amount of drug would be as follows:

$$100\% \ 50\% \ 25\% \ 12.5\% \ 6.25\%$$

$$T_{1/2} \ T_{1/2} \ T_{1/2} \ T_{1/2}$$

So if $T_{1/2}$ for a drug was 12 hours, it would take 48 hours for the serum concentration to reduce to 6.25% of the original.

This would be used to calculate how long to withdraw a drug for in an overdose situation.

Loading dose

Loading doses are used to ensure that a drug achieves a clinically effective serum concentration quickly when treatment is needed to be effective quickly, an example would be when treating infection.

Amount of drug in the body = target concentration × volume of distribution

$$\text{Loading dose} = \text{amount of drug in the body}$$

$$\text{Bioavailability} \times \text{salt fraction}$$

Molecular weights

You will rarely see calculations in community pharmacy involving molecular weight but you may see them in hospital pharmacy and usually relating to electrolyte imbalances.

The molecular weight of a compound is the sum of all the atomic weights of the individual atoms in the molecules and is measured in grams. For example:

$$KBr \text{ is } 1 \times 39 \text{ (atomic weight of potassium)} + 79.9 \text{ (atomic weight of bromine)} = 118.9 \text{ g}$$

$$AICE_3 \text{ is } 1 \times 27 \text{ (atomic weight of aluminium)} + 3 \times 35.5 \text{ (35.5 isatomic weight of chlorine and there are three of them)} = 133.5 \text{ g}$$

Drugs and their salts

Many drugs come with different salts attached to the basic drug molecule. A common example is iron. It is important to not therefore assume that there is the same amount of iron in the different formulae:

Ferrous sulphate ($FeSO_4$) has molecular weight of 152 g and contains 56 g of iron

Ferrous fumarate ($C_{12}H_{22}FeO_{12}.2H_2O$) has a molecular weight of 482 g but also contains 56 g of iron.

In practice this means that the weights of iron tablets do not indicate how much iron is in each tablet.

How many moles of individual ions are in a product?

If a solution contains 1 mole of KCl and 1 mole of NaCl, then we also have

1   mole of potassium ions

1   mole of sodium ions

2   moles of chloride ions (as we get a mole from each compound)

If a solution contains 1 mole of $CaCl_2$, then we also have

1   mole of calcium ions

2   moles of chloride ions (from the formula)

Key points

- Units are very important both in terms of size and system and you need to ensure you are familiar with the differences between them

- Answers should be 'sense' checked that they are appropriate for the patient in the situation described
- Strengths can be described in a variety of ways which relate to how the product was made
- Rounding should be used to make amounts practical to both supply and administer
- It is important to check the units of individual doses
- The quantity supplied needs to be calculated as accurately as any other pharmacy calculation
- Dilutions can be single- or multi-stage calculations
- When an amount of drug is administered intravenously over a period of time, this is described as an infusion rate
- If the patient has renal impairment, the amount of drug or frequency of administration may need to be adjusted
- Pharmacokinetic calculations are designed to ensure the clinical effectiveness of the drug is maximized whilst minimizing the risk of side-effects

Chapter | 2 |

Dispensing techniques (compounding and good practice)

Judith A. Rees

STUDY POINTS

- Practical aspects of dispensing
- The working environment and procedures
- Extemporaneous dispensing equipment and its correct use
- Manipulative techniques used in dispensing and compounding
- Ingredients and their selection
- Problem-solving in extemporaneous dispensing

Introduction

This chapter deals with some of the practical aspects of dispensing, concentrating on the small-scale manufacture of medicines from basic ingredients. This process is called *compounding* or *extemporaneous dispensing*. Additionally, good practice which applies to all aspects of dispensing will be considered.

Nowadays, most medicines are manufactured by the pharmaceutical industry under well-controlled conditions and packaged in suitable containers designed to maintain the stability of the product (e.g. sealed in an inert atmosphere). Extemporaneous dispensing, which cannot be as well-controlled, should only be used when a manufactured product is unavailable. Reasons for unavailability of products may include:

- Non-licensed products
- Products no longer on the market or unavailable from the manufacturer

- Products requiring an individualized dose, e.g. for paediatric or geriatric patients
- Products requiring an individualized formulation for a patient, e.g. the removal of colouring agents
- Veterinary products, e.g. formulations for different species.

The pharmacist undertaking extemporaneous dispensing has a responsibility to maintain equipment in working order, to ensure that the formula and dose are safe and appropriate and that all materials are sourced from recognized pharmaceutical manufacturers. There are also requirements concerning calculations, maintaining good records and labelling. Any staff involved in the process should be adequately trained. These requirements should all be incorporated within standard operating procedures (SOPs).

In any dispensing process, the end-product will be used or taken by a person or an animal. Therefore it is important that the medicine produced is of the highest achievable quality. This, in turn, means that the highest standards must be applied during the preparation process.

The working environment and procedures

Organization

The working environment needs to be organized, with well trained, efficient staff. A safe system of working is essential for a dispensary and the development and use of SOPs should be followed. Additionally, health and safety regulations must be applied in the dispensary.

Cleanliness and hygiene

The dispensing bench, the equipment, utensils and the container which is to hold the final product must all be clean. Lack of cleanliness can cause contamination of the preparation with other ingredients. For example, a spatula which has been used to remove an ingredient from one container will adulterate subsequent containers if not washed before being used again. Cleanliness will also minimize microbial contamination.

Dispensing staff should have a high standard of hygiene and hand-washing facilities should be readily available. A clean overall or uniform should be worn, hair tied back and, preferably, be covered with a disposable hat/cap and any skin lesions covered with a dressing. Disposable gloves should be worn during preparative work and discarded afterwards. Consideration should be given to the use of masks if volatile substances or fine powders are to be handled.

Documenting procedures and results

Keeping comprehensive records is an essential part of the dispensing process. Records must be kept for a minimum of 2 years (ideally 5 years) and include the formula and any calculations, the ingredients and quantities used, their sources, batch numbers and expiry date. All calculations or weights/volumes should be checked by two people and recorded. Any substances requiring special handling techniques or hazardous substances should be recorded with the precautions taken. The record for a prescribed item should also include the patient and prescription details and date of dispensing. A record must be kept of the personnel involved, including the responsible pharmacist. Any deviations from a SOP should be recorded.

Equipment

Not only is the selection of the correct equipment for the job essential, but the equipment must be used in the correct way and maintained in good order.

Weighing equipment

Weighing equipment can be divided into non-automatic and automatic weighing equipment. Non-automatic weighing equipment requires an operator to place and/ or remove the items from the balance pan. Such weighing equipment can be a mechanical beam balance, which has a pan on one end of the beam for weights and a pan on the other end of the beam for the material to be weighed (Fig. 2.1) or it can be an electronic top-pan balance, in which case the substance to be weighed is placed on the pan and an electronic display gives the weight. Automatic weighing equipment is designed to automatically fill a package to the required

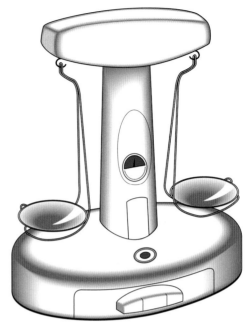

Fig. 2.1 Dispensing balance.

weight without the intervention of an operator. Such equipment is used in the pharmaceutical industry, and nowadays for extemporaneous dispensing. Whichever type of weighing equipment is used, it must be suitable for its intended use and be sufficiently accurate. In the UK, weighing equipment must be calibrated in metric units and must be marked with maximum and minimum weights that can be weighed.

General rules for the use and maintenance of weighing equipment

The following points are important to ensure accurate weighing:
- Balances must be placed on a level surface; most will incorporate a level indicator device to allow adjustment for a non-level surface
- Balances' readings must indicate zero before use. If zero is not indicated, then incorrect readings, and hence weights, may be obtained
- Strong draughts, caused by air conditioning or a breeze, can affect some balances and make a correct reading impossible. Therefore always site a balance in a draught-free area
- Always keep the balance pan clean and free from debris
- Regular checks with stamped weights should be made to ensure the balance is working correctly
- If possible, keep a record of when, and by whom, the check was carried out as well as the result
- Never weigh less than the declared minimum weight or more than the maximum weight declared on the balance

- Do not weigh ingredients on a piece of paper, as this introduces a potential inaccuracy. The exception is when weighing greasy or semi-solid materials, e.g. white soft paraffin, when a counterbalanced piece of paper should be used
- Always read the manufacturer's instructions before using an electronic balance
- Use tweezers to handle weights, if used. Never handle weights, as this will affect their accuracy and risks contamination.

Measuring liquids

Liquid measures

All measures for liquids must comply with current weights and measures regulations and should be stamped accordingly. Traditionally, conical measures (Fig. 2.2) have been used in dispensing.

When using a measure always ensure the following:

- The level of liquid is read to the bottom of the meniscus at eye level
- The measure is vertical when reading the meniscus. If this is not done, considerable errors in quantities can occur
- The measure is thoroughly drained to deliver the correct volume
- Always select the smallest measure which will hold the desired volume because this gives the greatest accuracy
- If the substance being measured is so viscous that it would be very difficult to drain the measure effectively, then the volume should be measured by difference. This is done by pouring an excess into the measure and then pouring off the liquid until only the excess volume remains.

Measuring small volumes

Graduated pipettes can be used for small volumes from 5 mL down to 0.1 mL. For volumes smaller than this, a dilution should be made. The viscosity of the substance being measured should also be considered.

Correct use of pipettes

Pipettes can be either the 'drainage' or 'blow-out' variety. A rubber bulb or teat should be used. Never use mouth suction.

- A bulb or teat should be placed over the mouth of the pipette
- Only a short length of the pipette should be immersed in the liquid
- The correct amount of liquid should be drawn up the pipette
- The measured liquid is then released into the desired container.

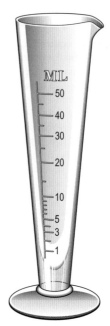

Fig. 2.2 Conical dispensing measure.

Nowadays, semi-automatic pipettes can be used for dispensing.

Mixing and grinding

Mortar and pestle

The mortar (bowl) and pestle (pounding device) are used to reduce the size of powders, mix powders, mix together powders and liquids and to make emulsions. Two types, each available in a range of sizes, are used.

Glass mortar and pestle

These are generally small. The smooth surface of the glass reduces the friction which can be generated, so they are only suitable for size reduction of friable materials (such as crystals). Glass mortars and pestles are useful for mixing small quantities of fine powders and for the mixing of substances such as dyes which are absorbed by and stain composition or porcelain mortars.

Porcelain or composition mortars and pestles

These mortars have a rough surface. They are ideal for size reduction of solids and for mixing solids and liquids, as in the preparation of suspensions and emulsions.

Size reduction using a mortar and pestle

Selection of the correct type of mortar and pestle is vital for this operation. A flat-bottomed mortar and a pestle with a flat head should be chosen.

Using a mortar and pestle for mixing powders

Adequate mixing will only be achieved if there is sufficient space. Overfilling of the mortar should be avoided. The pestle should be rotated in both right and left directions to ensure thorough mixing. Undue pressure should not be used, as this will cause impaction of the powder on the bottom of the mortar.

Filters

There are occasions when clarification of a liquid is required. Where filtration is required, filter paper or membrane filters should be used. Filter paper and membrane filters come in different grades and selection of the correct grade is determined by the size of the particles to be removed. Filter paper has the disadvantage of introducing fibres into the filtrate and may also absorb significant amounts of active ingredient. This is less likely with membrane filters.

Heat sources

In the dispensing process, it may be necessary to heat ingredients, e.g. melt semi-solids in the preparation of ointments/creams, warm liquids to aid dissolution of solids.

Nowadays, water baths or electrically heated hot plates are used for heating.

Manipulative techniques

Selection of the correct equipment and using it appropriately is fundamental to good compounding. Several basic manipulative techniques may require practice.

Mixing

The goal of any mixing operation should be to ensure even distribution of all the ingredients has occurred. If a sample is removed from any part of the final preparation, it should be identical to a sample taken from any other part of the container.

Mixing of liquids

Simple stirring or shaking is usually all that is required to mix two or more liquids. The degree of stirring or shaking will be dependent on the viscosities of the liquids.

Mixing solids with liquids

Particle size reduction will either speed up the dissolution process or improve the uniform distribution of the solid throughout the liquid. When a solution is being made, a stirring rod will be adequate. However, a suspension will require a mortar and pestle.

Mixing solids with solids

Where the quantity of material to be mixed is small and the proportions are approximately the same, the materials can be added to an appropriately sized mortar and effectively mixed. Where a small quantity of powder has to be mixed with a large quantity, in order to achieve effective mixing, it must be done in stages:

*   The ingredient with the smallest bulk is placed in the mortar
*   A quantity of the second ingredient, approximately equal in volume to the first, is added and carefully mixed, using the pestle
*   A further quantity of the second ingredient, approximately equal in volume to the mixture in the mortar, is now added
*   This process, known as 'doubling-up', is continued until all the powder has been added (see Ch. 10).

Mixing semi-solids

If all the ingredients are semi-solids or liquids, they can be mixed together by rubbing them down on an ointment slab, using a spatula. If there is a significant difference in the quantities of the ingredients, a 'doubling-up' process should be used. An alternative method is the fusion method.

The fusion method

*   Place the bases in an evaporating basin and gently heat until they have just melted. Excess heat should not be used, as overheating may cause physical or chemical changes in some materials
*   The basin is then removed from the heat and the contents are stirred continuously, but gently, until the mixture has cooled and set. Stirring at this stage is of vital importance as otherwise the components may segregate on cooling. Rapid stirring should be avoided as it will introduce air bubbles into the mixture.

When using the fusion method, do not be tempted to add any solid active ingredients to the basin before the bases have set. Addition of any further ingredients is best done by rubbing down on an ointment slab. (Further details of methods used in the preparation of ointments can be found in Ch. 8.)

Tared containers

Liquid preparations should, as far as possible, be made up to volume in a measure. There are, however, instances when accurate transfer of the preparation to the final container is difficult, e.g. with some suspensions it can be almost impossible to remove all the insoluble ingredients when pouring from one container to another. Emulsions and viscous preparations can also be difficult to transfer accurately. In these cases, a tared container should be used.

To tare a bottle

A volume of potable water identical to the volume of the product being dispensed is accurately measured. This is then poured into the chosen medicine container and the meniscus marked with the upper edge of a small adhesive label, effectively making the bottle into a single-point measure. The container is then emptied and allowed to drain thoroughly. The preparation is then poured into the container and made up to volume, using the tare mark as the guide. Remove the tare label.

Ingredients

All ingredients must be sourced and obtained from reputable suppliers and be of a quality suitable for the preparation and dispensing of pharmaceutical products. Additionally, ingredients must be suitably stored to preserve stability and integrity. For example, regular checks on expiry dates of stored products should be made and any ingredient outside its expiry date should be discarded. Some ingredients may require special storage conditions and these should be provided. Many pharmaceutical ingredients and products require storage in a refrigerator, which should be fitted with a maximum/minimum thermometer and both maximum and minimum temperatures checked and recorded on a daily basis.

Selection

When dispensing, selection of the correct product is vital. The label on each container must be read carefully and checked to ensure that it contains the required product. There are many examples of drugs and preparations where names may be misread if care is not taken; examples include folic acid and folinic acid, cefuroxime and cefotaxime.

Variety of forms

Some ingredients of extemporaneously dispensed medicines may occur in a variety of forms or a synonym is used. Coal tar, for example, is available as coal tar solution, strong coal tar solution and coal tar. Some other materials

Table 2.1 Some substances which occur in a variety of forms

Substance/form	Use
Light magnesium carbonate	Because of its lightness and diffusible properties, it is used in suspensions
Heavy magnesium carbonate	Normally used in bulk or individual powders
Light kaolin	Used in suspensions
Heavy kaolin	Used in the preparation of kaolin poultice
Precipitated sulphur	This has a smaller particle size than sublimed sulphur and is preferred in preparations for external use, e.g. suspensions, creams and ointments
Sublimed sulphur	Slightly gritty powder, which does not produce such elegant preparations as precipitated sulphur
Yellow soft paraffin	Used as an ointment base
White soft paraffin	Bleached yellow soft paraffin, normally used when the other ingredients are not strongly coloured

where confusion can occur are listed in Table 2.1. This list is not meant to be comprehensive and only contains common exemplars. To reduce the risk of errors, you need to read the container label carefully and have it checked by a second person.

Problem-solving in extemporaneous dispensing

For extemporaneous dispensing, it is helpful if a method detailing how to prepare the product is available. Methods for 'official' preparations can sometimes be found in reference sources such as the *Pharmaceutical Codex*. However, on many occasions, no method is available. In such a situation, it may be helpful to consider similar formulas in reference sources. Additionally, the application of simple scientific knowledge, especially of physical properties, is often all that is needed. The following gives an example of how this is done.

Putting theory into practice
Solubility

Always check the solubility of any solid materials. If they are soluble in the main vehicles, then a solution is likely to be produced. If solubility is limited to one liquid, this will assist in achieving uniform dose distribution. Solution will be achieved more quickly if the particle size is small and so size reduction should be considered for any soluble ingredients which are presented in a lumpy or granular form. It is also necessary to add less soluble solids before more soluble solids. If the substance is not soluble, then a suspension will need to be produced. Whether a suspending agent will be required should be considered (see Ch. 6). Where one material is an oil and another aqueous, it is likely that an emulsifying agent will be required to produce an emulsion (see Ch. 7).

Volatile ingredients

If an ingredient is volatile, then it should be added near the end of the dispensing process and often directly into the final container. If it is added too early, much may be lost due to evaporation.

Viscosity

The viscosity of a liquid will have a bearing on how it is measured, i.e. is a pipette or measure suitable, or should it be measured by difference, and how will it be incorporated?

Expiry date

All extemporaneously prepared products should be labelled with an expiry date. Ideally, stability studies should be undertaken in order to predict an accurate shelf-life for all products. This is not usually possible for 'one-off' preparations and most hospital pharmacies have guidelines based on previous stability studies. If in doubt, use the shortest possible expiry date, e.g. 3 days, and be prepared to produce the medicine in small quantities every 3 days.

Conclusion

Developing good practice in dispensing takes time and requires attention to detail.

Key points

- Extemporaneous dispensing should only be used when manufactured medicines are not available
- Accurate dispensing requires clean and methodical work
- Always comply with SOPs
- Comprehensive records of extemporaneous dispensing are required to be kept for at least 2 years
- Always use all equipment correctly
- Ensure that liquid measures comply with the weights and measures regulations
- Always use the bottom of the meniscus when measuring liquids
- Viscous liquids should be measured 'by difference'
- Select the smallest measure or pipette for the volume of liquid to be measured
- A glass mortar and pestle can be used for size reduction of friable materials and mixing small quantities of fine powder
- A porcelain mortar and pestle is used for larger quantities, for mixing solids and liquids, making emulsions and for size reduction
- Confusion can arise with different forms of the same material and the use of synonyms
- Simple problem-solving techniques can produce a satisfactory method of dispensing a product

Chapter 3

Oral unit dosage forms

Arthur J. Winfield

STUDY POINTS

- Different types of tablets
- Excipients used in tablets and capsules
- Dispensing commercially produced tablets and capsules
- Extemporaneous dispensing of capsules and cachets

Introduction

Tablets and capsules (oral unit dosage forms) are the most popular way of delivering a drug for oral use. They are convenient for the patient and are usually easy to handle and identify. They are produced by the pharmaceutical industry, where quality assurance ensures a high accuracy of dose within each individual dosage form. They are free from the problems of stability found in aqueous mixtures and suspensions. Packaging in blister packs can also enhance the stability of these dosage forms. The main disadvantages are that there is a slower onset of action relative to liquids and some people have difficulty swallowing solid oral dosage forms, e.g. the very young or very old.

Tablets

Tablets are solid preparations each containing a single dose of one or more active ingredient(s). They are normally prepared by compressing uniform volumes of particles, although some tablets are prepared by moulding.

Many different types of tablet are available, which may be in a variety of shapes and sizes. The types include dispersible, effervescent, chewable, sublingual and buccal tablets, lozenges, tablets for rectal or vaginal administration and solution tablets. Some tablets are designed to release the drug after a time lag, or slowly for a prolonged drug release or sustained drug action (see Ch. 19). The design of these modified-release tablets uses formulation techniques to control the biopharmaceutical behaviour of the drug. In addition to the drug(s), several excipients must be added. These will aid the process of tableting and ensure that the active ingredient will be released as intended. Excipients include:

- *Diluents.* These add bulk to make the tablet easier to handle. Examples include lactose, mannitol, sorbitol and calcium carbonate
- *Binders.* These enable granules to be prepared which improves the flow properties of the mixture during manufacture. Examples include polyvinylpyrrolidone and microcrystalline cellulose
- *Disintegrants.* These encourage the tablet to break into smaller particles after ingestion. Examples include modified cellulose and modified starch
- *Lubricants, glidants, antiadherents.* These are essential for the flow of the tablet material into the tablet dies and preventing sticking of the compressed tablet in the punch and die. Examples of lubricants are magnesium and calcium stearate, sodium lauryl sulphate and sodium stearyl fumarate. Colloidal silica is usually the glidant of choice. Talc and magnesium stearate are effective antiadherents
- *Miscellaneous agents* may be added, such as colours and flavours in chewable tablets.

Some tablets have coatings, such as sugar coating or film coating. Coatings can protect the tablet from environmental damage, mask an unpleasant taste, aid identification of the tablet and enhance its appearance. Enteric (gastro-resistant) coatings on tablets resist dissolution or disruption of the tablet in the stomach, but not in the intestine. This is useful when a drug is destroyed by gastric acid, is irritating to the gastric mucosa or, when bypassing the stomach, aids drug absorption.

Dispensing of tablets

Many tablets in the UK and other countries are packaged by the manufacturer into patient packs suitable for issue to the patient without repacking by the pharmacist. Patient information leaflets are also contained in these patient packs. When dispensing these packs to patients, the pharmacist must ensure that they are labelled correctly, according to the prescriber's instructions, and that the patient is counselled on the use of the medication.

For some controlled-release tablets, variations in bioavailability may occur with different brands. It is important that patients are given the brand that they are stabilized on in order to maintain therapeutic outcome. Examples where this is important include theophylline, lithium and phenytoin.

Tablets may also be supplied in a bulk container. The required number of tablets needs to be counted out (see Ch. 2) and placed in a suitable container for dispensing to the patient (see Ch. 4). It is important to minimize errors by ensuring that the correct bulk container has been selected and the correct drug dispensed. The pharmacist should verify this by checking the label of the bulk container and by examining the shape, size and markings on the dispensed tablets where appropriate, with the prescription. A copy of the patient information leaflet should be included.

Some tablets are supplied in a strip-packed form where each tablet has its own blister. A development of this is the calendar pack where the day or date on which the tablet is to be taken is indicated on the pack.

Shelf-life and storage of tablets

Most tablets should be stored in airtight packaging, protected from light and extremes of temperature. When stored properly, they generally have a long shelf-life. The expiry date will be printed on the package or the individual strip packs. Some tablets need to be stored in a cool place, e.g. Ketovite and Leukeran (chlorambucil) (both stored between 2 and 8°C). Some tablets contain volatile drugs, e.g. glyceryl trinitrate, and must be packed in glass containers with tightly fitting metal screw caps (see Ch. 4).

Containers for tablets

Strip or blister packs are dispensed in a paperboard box and tablets counted from bulk containers are placed in

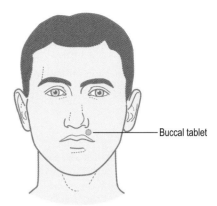

Fig. 3.1 Positioning of a buccal tablet.

amber glass or plastic containers with airtight, child-resistant closures.

Special labels and advice on tablets

Most tablets should be swallowed with a glass, or 'draught', of water. A draught of water refers to a volume of water of about 50 mL. This prevents the dosage from becoming lodged in the oesophagus, which can cause problems such as ulceration. Tablets may be coated and shaped to aid swallowing.

Some tablets should be dissolved or dispersed in water before taking, e.g. effervescent tablets. Other tablets, particularly those with coatings or modified-release properties, should be swallowed whole. There are also some tablets which should be chewed or sucked before swallowing. Appropriate labels should be placed on the container.

Coated tablets, e.g. enteric (gastro-resistant) coatings, require specific advice on avoiding indigestion remedies at the same time of day, as these will affect the pH of the stomach, and therefore cause premature breakdown of the enteric coating on the tablet.

Buccal and sublingual tablets are not swallowed whole because they will not have their intended therapeutic effect. Figure 3.1 illustrates the positioning for buccal tablets. Sublingual tablets are placed under the tongue.

Capsules

Capsules are solid preparations intended for oral administration made with a hard or soft gelatin shell. One (or more) medicament is enclosed within this gelatin container. Most capsules are swallowed whole, but some contain granules which provide a useful pre-measured dose for administering in a similar way to a powder, e.g. formulations of pancreatin. Some capsules enclose enteric-coated pellets, e.g. Erymax (erythromycin). Capsules are elegant, easy to swallow and can be useful in masking unpleasant tastes. Capsules may also be used to hold oils for inhalation, e.g. Karvol or for rectal and vaginal administration, e.g. Gyno-Daktarin (miconazole nitrate) (see Ch. 9).

Soft shell capsules

A soft gelatin capsule consists of a flexible solid shell containing powders, non-aqueous liquids, solutions, emulsions, suspensions or pastes. Such capsules allow liquids to be given as solid dosage forms, e.g. cod-liver oil. They also offer accurate dosage, improved stability and overcome some of the problems of dealing with powders. They are formed, filled and sealed in one manufacturing process.

Hard shell capsules

Empty capsule shells are made from gelatin and are clear, colourless and essentially tasteless. Colourings and markings can be easily added for light protection and to ease identification. The shells are used in the preparation of most manufactured capsules and for the extemporaneous compounding of capsules. The shell comprises two sections, the body and the cap, both being cylindrical and sealed at one end. Powder or particulate solid, such as granules and pellets, can be placed in the body and the capsule closed by bringing the body and cap together (Fig. 3.2). Some capsules have small indentations on the body and cap which 'lock' together.

Compounding of capsules

Occasionally hand filling of capsules may be required, particularly in a hospital pharmacy or when preparing materials for clinical trials. A suitable size of capsule shell should be selected so that the finished capsule looks reasonably full. Hard shell capsules are available in eight sizes. These are listed in Table 3.1, with the corresponding approximate capacity (based on lactose). The bulk density of a powder mixture will also affect the choice of capsule size.

Calculations for compounding capsules

The recommended minimum weight for filling a capsule is 100 mg. If the required weight of the drug is smaller than this, a diluent should be added by trituration (see Ch. 10). If the quantity of the drug for a batch of capsules is smaller than the minimum weighable amount, 100 mg on a Class B balance, then trituration will also be required. Lactose and starch are commonly used diluents. To allow for small

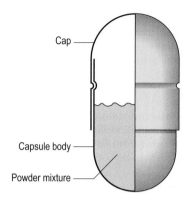

Fig. 3.2 Hard gelatin capsule shell: body and cap.

losses of powder, an excess should be calculated, e.g. two extra capsules (see Ch. 10).

Filling capsules

The number of capsules to be filled should be counted and set to one side. This avoids the danger of contaminating empty capsules. The powder to be encapsulated should be finely sifted (180 μm sieve) and prepared. Magnesium stearate (up to 1% weight in weight (w/w)) and silica may be added as a lubricant and glidant respectively, to aid filling of the capsule. Various methods of filling capsules on a small scale are possible.

Filling from a powder mass

The prepared powder can be placed on a clean tile or piece of demy paper and powder pushed into the capsule body with the aid of a spatula until the required weight has been enclosed. The empty capsule body could also be 'punched' into a heap of powder until filled. Alternatively, create a small funnel from demy paper and fill the capsule body with the required weight. Gloves should be worn to protect the capsules from handling.

Filling with weighed aliquots

Weighed aliquots of powder may be placed on paper and channelled into the empty capsule shell. A sharp fold in the paper helps direct the powder. Alternatively, simple apparatus is available for small-scale manufacture of larger numbers of capsules. A plastic plate with rows of cavities to hold the empty capsule bodies is used, different rows holding different sizes of capsules. A plastic bridge containing a row of holes corresponding to the position of the capsule cavities can then be used to support a long-stemmed funnel. The end of the funnel passes into the mouth of the capsule below. The stem of the funnel should be as wide as possible for the size of the capsule to assist with powder

Table 3.1 Sizes of hard gelatin capsules and their approximate capacities

Capsule no.	000	00	0	1	2	3	4	5
Content (mg)	950	650	450	300	250	200	150	100

flow. A weighed aliquot of powder can then be poured into the capsule via the funnel. A thin plastic rod or wire may be used to 'tamp' the powder to break blockages or to lightly compress the material inside the capsule. After filling the capsule, the cap can be fitted loosely and the weight checked before sealing.

Capsules are subject to tests for uniformity of weight and content of active ingredient, and uniformity of content where the content of active ingredient is <2 mg or <2% by weight of the total capsule fill.

Shelf-life and storage of capsules

If stability data are not available for extemporaneously filled capsules, then a short expiry date (up to 4 weeks) should be given. Manufactured capsules will be assigned expiry dates on the container and the packed strips or blister packs. Most capsules need to be stored in a cool, dry place.

Containers for capsules

The containers used for capsules are similar to those for tablets. Some capsules are susceptible to moisture absorption and desiccants may be included in the packaging.

Special labels and advice on capsules

Capsules should be swallowed whole with a glass of water or other liquid. Advice may be sought from the pharmacist about whether it is acceptable to empty the contents of a capsule onto food or into water for ease of swallowing. In giving this advice, the release characteristics of the dosage form should be considered; for instance, whether it is an enteric-coated or prolonged-release formulation.

Other oral unit dosage forms

Pastilles

These contain a glycerol and gelatine base. They are sweetened, flavoured and medicated and are popular over-the-counter remedies for soothing coughs and sore throats.

Example 3.1 Prepare eight capsules each containing haloperidol 10 mg and 1% w/w magnesium stearate.

	For 1 capsule	For 10 capsules
Haloperidol	10 mg	100 mg
Magnesium stearate	1 mg	10 mg
Lactose	89 mg	890 mg

Formulation notes. Magnesium stearate is added to act as a lubricant to aid flow of the powder into the capsule; 10 mg is not weighable, so a trituration must be carried out. Lactose acts as a diluent to bring the weight of each capsule fill to 100 mg.

Trituration for magnesium stearate:

Magnesium stearate	100 mg
Lactose	900 mg

Take a 100 mg portion of this mixture, which will contain 10 mg of magnesium stearate and 90 mg of lactose.

Method of preparation. Sieve the powders using a 180 m sieve. Prepare the magnesium stearate triturate. Weigh 100 mg of haloperidol, and mix this with the magnesium stearate triturate in a mortar and pestle. Gradually add 800 mg of lactose to this mixture, by doubling-up. This gives a total powder quantity of 1000 mg (equivalent to 10 100 mg capsules). Fill the capsule shells (size 4 or 5) with 100 mg aliquots, checking the weight of each capsule before sealing. Pack eight capsules in an amber glass or plastic tablet container with a child-resistant closure.

Storage and shelf-life. Store in a cool, dry place and protect from light. Expiry date of 2 weeks, since stability in capsule form is unknown.

Key points

- Tablets and capsules are the most common dosage forms
- Excipients are added to improve manufacture, handling and release of the drug

- Tablets and capsules should be swallowed normally with about 50 mL of water
- Some tablets are designed to be chewed, dissolved, swallowed whole or delivered by the buccal or sublingual route
- Tablets cannot be made extemporaneously, but capsules are filled when preparing for clinical trials

- Capsule size is selected so that they look reasonably full
- The minimum weight of contents in an extemporaneous capsule is 100 mg
- Medicated glycerol-gelatin-based pastilles are popular for coughs and sore throats

Chapter | 4 |

Packaging

Derek G. Chapman

STUDY POINTS

- Definition of a container
- Considerations made in selecting a container
- The difference between primary and secondary packaging
- The materials used for packaging, including glass, plastics, metal and paper
- Types of container in common use
- Child-resistant closures and tamper-evident seals
- Patient pack dispensing

Introduction

Pharmaceutical formulations must be suitably contained, protected and labelled from the time of manufacture until the patient uses them. Throughout this period, the container must maintain the quality, safety and stability of the medicine and protect the product against physical, climatic, chemical and biological hazards. The *British Pharmacopoeia* identifies the closure as part of the container.

To promote good patient compliance, the container must be user-friendly. Thus containers should be easy to open and reclose, most notably for elderly or arthritic patients. Other factors must also be considered in the selection of the container used to package a pharmaceutical formulation, including the cost and the need for both child-resistant closures and tamper-evident seals.

Repackaging may be performed for dispensing purposes in the community and hospital pharmacies and in specialized production facilities (see Chs 2 and 3). Bulk medicines are repackaged into smaller quantities in dispensing containers for distribution to hospital wards, clinics and general practitioners for direct supply to patients. This is mostly carried out with tablets and capsules that are transferred from bulk quantities into smaller amounts that are more suitable for patient use. In the UK, this process is performed in the hospital pharmacy where the MHRA allows the repackaging of small batches of up to 25 containers. Larger batches must be packed in licensed manufacturing premises. The facilities used for these repackaging operations are designed to maintain the quality of the medicine.

The composition of containers and closures used for the repackaging of bulk medicines must be carefully selected and must be of a quality as good as the original container. Both glass and plastic containers are used for repackaging but glass containers are often preferred due to the more inert qualities of glass.

Primary containers used for repackaging must not:
- Allow product leakage
- Chemically react with the product
- Release components
- Absorb or adsorb the product components.

The container used in the repackaging process must protect the product from:
- Physical damage
- Chemical and microbial contamination
- Light, moisture and oxygen as appropriate.

As the medicine has been transferred into a new container, the expiry date of the repackaged medicine must not exceed 12 months, unless the stability of the repackaged product justifies a longer shelf-life. The details of these repackaging processes must be recorded.

Each container of the repackaged batch is labelled with the:
- Identity and quantity of the medicine
- Batch number
- Appropriate storage instructions
- Product expiry date
- Requirements for handling and storage.

There are some situations where the repackaging is limited, such as with glyceryl trinitrate tablets, owing to the potential loss of the volatile drug (see Ch. 3). Sterile products cannot easily be repackaged and require effective closure systems to minimize the risk of microbial contamination of the contents within the container. In addition, the pack itself must withstand sterilization procedures. Consequently, care must be applied to the selection of the container and its closure for the packaging of sterile products (see also Chs 11, 12, 15 and 17).

Primary and secondary packaging

Primary packaging materials are in direct contact with the product. This also applies to the closure, which is also part of the primary pack. It is important that this container must not interact with the medicine. It must protect the medicine from damage and from extraneous chemical and microbial contamination. In addition, the primary packaging should support the use of the product by the patient. Secondary packages are additional packaging materials that improve the appearance of the product and include outer wrappers or labels that do not make direct contact with the product (Table 4.1). Secondary packages can also supply information about the product and its use. They should provide evidence of tampering with the medicine.

The following terms are used to describe containers:

Single-dose containers hold the medicine that is intended for single use. For example, a glass ampoule

Multidose containers hold a quantity of the material that will be used as two or more doses. For example, a multiple dose vial or a plastic tablet bottle

Well-closed containers protect the product from contamination with unwanted foreign materials and from loss of contents during use

Airtight containers are impermeable to solids, liquids and gases during normal storage and use. If the container is to be opened on more than one occasion it must remain airtight after re-closure

Sealed containers such as glass ampoules are closed by fusion of the container material

Tamper-evident containers are closed containers fitted with a device that irreversibly indicates if the container has been opened

Light-resistant containers protect the contents from the effect of radiation at a wavelength between 290 nm and 450 nm

Child-resistant containers, commonly referred to as *CRCs*, are designed to prevent children accessing the potentially hazardous product

Strip packs have at least one sealed pocket of material with each pocket containing a single dose of the product. The pack is made of two layers of film or laminate material. The nature and the level of protection that is required by the contained product will affect the composition of these layers

Blister packs are composed of a base layer, with cavities that contain the pharmaceutical product, and a lid. This lid is sealed to the base layer by heat, pressure or both. They are more rigid than strip packs and are not used for powders or semi-solids. Blister packs can be printed with day and week identifiers to produce calendar packs. These identifiers will support patient compliance

Tropicalized packs are blister packs with an additional aluminium membrane to provide greater protection against high humidity

Pressurized packs expel the product through a valve. The pressure for the expulsion of the product is provided by the positive pressure of the propellant that is often a compressed or liquefied gas (see Ch. 14)

Original packs are pharmaceutical packs that are commercially produced and intended for finite treatment periods. These packs are dispensed directly to the patient in their original form. Manufacturer's information is contained on the pack but the pharmacist must attach a dispensing label.

An important consideration when selecting the packaging for any product is that its main objective is that the package must contribute to delivering a drug to a specific site of effective activity in the patient.

Table 4.1 Types of primary and secondary packaging materials and their use

Material	Type	Examples of use
Glass	Primary	Metric medical bottle, ampoule, vial
Plastic	Primary	Ampoule, vial, container, infusion fluid dropper bottle
Plastic	Secondary	Wrapper to contain primary pack
Board	Secondary	Box to contain primary pack
Paper	Secondary	Labels, patient information leaflet

The selection of packaging for a pharmaceutical product is dependent on the following factors:

- The nature of the product itself: its chemical activity, sensitivity to moisture and oxygen, compatibility with packaging materials
- The type of patient: is it to be used by an elderly or arthritic patient or by a child?
- The dosage form
- Method of administering the medication
- Required shelf-life
- Product use.

Packaging materials

Glass

Historically, glass has been widely used as a drug packaging material. It continues to be the preferred packaging material for many pharmaceutical products.

Glass does have several advantages:

- It is inert to most medicinal products
- It is impervious to air and moisture
- It allows easy inspection of the container's contents
- It can be coloured to protect contents from harmful wavelengths of light
- It is easy to clean and sterilize by heat
- It is available in variously shaped containers.
The disadvantages of glass include:
- It is fragile: glass fragments can be released into the product during transport or contaminants can penetrate the product by way of cracks in the container
- Certain types of glass release alkali into the container contents
- It is expensive when compared with the price of plastic
- It is heavy, resulting in increased transport costs.

The chemical stability of glass for pharmaceutical use is given by the resistance of the glass to the release of soluble minerals into water contacting the glass. This is known as the *hydrolytic resistance*. Details are given in the *British Pharmacopoeia* (2012) for three types of glass.

Type I glass

This is also known as *neutral glass* or *borosilicate glass*. It possesses a high hydrolytic resistance due to the chemical composition of the glass. It is the most inert type of pharmaceutical glass with the lowest coefficient of thermal expansion. As a result, it is unlikely to crack on exposure to rapid temperature changes. Type I glass is suitable for packing all pharmaceutical preparations. However, it is expensive and this restricts its applications. It is widely used as glass ampoules and vials to package fluids for injection. In addition, it is used to package solutions that could dissolve

basic oxides in the glass. This would increase the pH of the formulation and could affect the drug stability and potency.

Type II glass

This is made of soda-lime-silica glass with a high hydrolytic resistance due to surface treatment of the glass. Type II glass is used to package aqueous preparations. In general, it is not used by manufacturers to package parenteral formulations with a pH <7. It is the glass used to produce containers for eye preparations and other dropper bottles.

Type III glass

This is made of a soda-lime-silica glass. It has a similar composition to Type II glass but contains more leachable oxides. It is commonly used to produce dispensary metric medical bottles. It is also suitable for packaging non-aqueous parenteral products and powders for injection.

Types of glass containers

Bottles

These are commonly used in the dispensary as amber metric medical bottles and are available in sizes from 50 mL to 500 mL supplied with a screw closure.

Amber metric medical bottles have a smooth curved side and a flat side (Fig. 4.1).

Dropper bottles

Eye drop and dropper bottles for ear and nasal use are hexagonal-shaped amber glass containers fluted on three sides. They are fitted with a cap, rubber teat and dropper as the

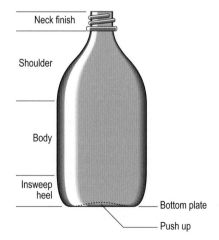

Neck finish

Shoulder

Body

Insweep heel

Bottom plate

Push up

Fig. 4.1 Metric medicine bottle.

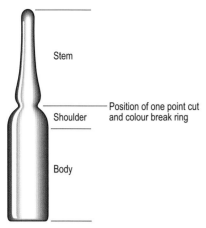

Fig. 4.2 Glass ampoule.

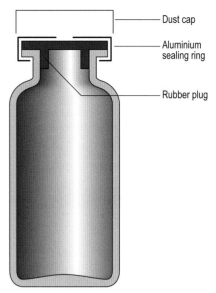

Fig. 4.3 Glass vial.

closure. The bottles are used at a capacity of 10 mL or 20 mL. The label is attached to the plain sides of the bottle.

Jars

Powders and semi-solid preparations are generally packed in wide-mouthed cylindrical jars made of clear or amber glass. The capacity of these jars varies from 15 mL to 500 mL. Ointment jars are used for packing extemporaneously prepared ointments and pastes. They are also used to repackage commercial products where microbial contamination by the patient's fingers is not detrimental to the product.

Containers for parenteral products

Small-volume parenteral products, such as subcutaneous injections, are typically packaged in various containers made of Type I glass. Glass ampoules (Fig. 4.2) are used to package parenteral solutions intended for single use.

Multiple-dose vials (Fig. 4.3) are used to package parenteral formulations that will be used on more than one occasion. Large-volume parenteral fluids have been packaged in 500 mL glass containers but these have been largely superseded by plastic bags.

Plastics

Plastics have been widely used for several years as containers for the product and as secondary packaging in the form of a carton. In more recent times, plastic has been developed for the packaging of parenteral products, including infusion fluids and small-volume injections.

Two classes of plastics are used in the packaging of pharmaceutical products. These are known as thermosets and thermoplastics. The thermosets are used for making screw caps for glass and metal containers. Thermoplastic polymers are used in the manufacture of a wide variety of pharmaceutical packages, as detailed in Table 4.2.

Table 4.2 The application of thermoplastic polymers for the packaging of pharmaceutical products

Polymer	Examples of application
High-density polyethylene	Solid dosage form containers
Low-density polyethylene	Flexible eye drop bottles
Linear low-density polyethylene	Heat-sealable containers
Polypropylene	Container closures, intravenous solution bottles
Polyvinyl chloride	Laminate for blister packs, intravenous bags
Polystyrene	Containers for oils and creams and solid dosage forms

The advantages of plastics for packaging are that:
- They release few particles into the product
- They are flexible and not easily broken
- They are of low density and thus light in weight
- They can be heat-sealed
- They are easily moulded into various shapes
- They are suitable for use as container, closure and as secondary packaging
- They are cheap.

The disadvantages of plastics are that:
- They are not as chemically inert as Type I glass
- Some plastics undergo stress cracking and distortion from contact with some chemicals

- Some plastics are very heat sensitive
- They are not as impermeable to gas and vapour as glass
- They may possess an electrostatic charge which will attract particles
- Additives in the plastic are easily leached into the product
- Substances such as the active drug and preservatives may be taken up from the product.

Plastic pharmaceutical containers are made of at least one polymer together with additives. The additives used will depend on the composition of the polymer and the production methods used.

Additives used in plastic containers include:

- Plasticizers
- Resins
- Stabilizers
- Lubricants
- Antistatic agents
- Mould-release agents.

Plastic containers

These are used for many types of pack, including rigid bottles for tablets and capsules, squeezable bottles for eye drops and nasal sprays, jars, flexible tubes, strip and blister packs. The composition and the physical shape of the containers vary widely to suit the application.

The principal plastic materials used in pharmaceutical packaging

Polyethylene
This is used as high- and low-density polyethylene, both of which are compatible with a wide range of drugs and are extensively used for the packaging of various pharmacy products. Of these two forms of polyethylene, low-density polyethylene (LDPE) is softer, more flexible and more easily stretched than high-density polyethylene (HDPE). Consequently, LDPE is usually the preferred plastic for squeeze bottles. By contrast, HDPE is stronger, stiffer, less clear, less permeable to gases and more resistant to oils, chemicals and solvents. It is commonly pigmented or printed white to block light transmission and improve label clarity. HDPE is widely used in bottles for solid dosage forms.

Disadvantages of LDPE and HDPE for packaging are that they:

- are softened by flavouring and aromatic oils
- are unsuitable for packing oxygen-sensitive products owing to high gas permeability
- adsorb antimicrobial preservative agents
- crack on contact with organic solvents.

Polyvinyl chloride (PVC)
This is extensively used as rigid packaging material and as the main component of intravenous bags.

Polypropylene
This is a strong, stiff plastic polymer with good resistance to cracking when flexed. As a result, it is particularly suitable for use in closures with hinges which must resist repeated flexing. In addition, polypropylene has been used as tablet containers and intravenous bottles.

Polystyrene
This is a clear, hard, brittle material with low impact resistance. Its use in drug packaging is limited due to its high permeability to water vapour. However, it has been used for tubes and amber-tinted bottles where clarity and stiffness are important and high gas permeability is not a drawback. It is also used for jars for ointments and creams with low water content.

Closures

Any closure system should provide an effective seal to retain the container contents and exclude external contaminants. CRCs commonly consist of a glass or plastic vial or bottle with a specially designed closure. These CRCs are a professional requirement for dispensing of solid and liquid dosage forms in the UK and are ultimately a compromise between child resistance and ease of opening. They are not an absolute barrier to children accessing medicine containers, therefore the containers should be stored in a safe place. Several designs of CRCs are currently used for pharmaceutical packaging, including cap–bottle alignment systems, push down and turn caps and, less commonly, squeeze and turn caps.

The closures in common use with dispensed medicines are the Snap-safe alignment closure (Fig. 4.4) and the push down and turn Clic-loc closure (Fig. 4.5). The Clic-loc child-resistant closures are based on the assumption that young children are unable to coordinate two separate and dissimilar actions; that is, applying pressure and rotating the closure top. The Clic-loc closure has a two-piece mechanism with springs between the inner and the outer parts. As a result of this design, the closure produces an audible clicking noise when the cap is turned without first being depressed. The inner cap is composed of polypropylene while the outer overcap is made of HDPE.

Contamination of the screw thread with crystallized sugar arising from syrups can increase the torque necessary to open these Clic-loc closures. This type of problem can restrict their suitability for use. Owing to opening difficulties experienced by some adults, these closures should not be used on containers supplied to elderly or disabled patients with poor manual dexterity. They should not be used when a request is made that the product is not dispensed with a CRC fitted. A Clic-loc closure must only

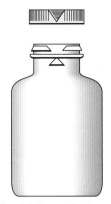

Fig. 4.4 Snap-safe closure.

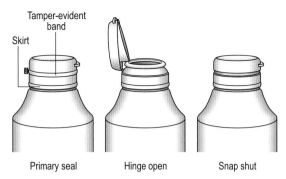

Fig. 4.6 Tamper-evident closure.

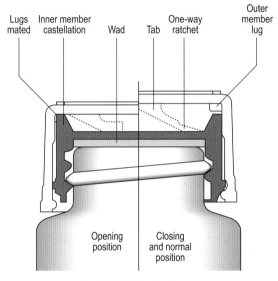

Fig. 4.5 Clic-loc® closure.

be dispensed on one occasion as continued use increases the penetration of moisture vapour into the container and decreases the child-resistant properties of the closure.

In recent years, greater awareness of the vulnerability of products has led to the development of tamper-evident closures. The closures indicate if unlawful access to the container contents has occurred and are currently available in various designs suitable for different containers and closures. Dispensary stock containers are frequently fitted with a Jaycap type of tamper-evident closure. These closures are made of either white polypropylene or LDPE. With this closure design, the tamper-evident closures snap over a security bead on the neck of the container. The closures cannot be opened until the tamper-evident band connecting the cap to the skirt is torn away (Fig. 4.6).

Clic-loc closures are available with this design, whereby an external tamper-evident coloured band must be removed before the closure can be turned. Tamper-evident inner seals are positioned within the closure and are attached to the rim of the opening to the container isolating its contents. The seal must be torn or removed from the container to gain access to the packaged product. These seals are commonly made of a combination of paper, plastic and foil.

Collapsible tubes

These are flexible containers for the storage and dispensing of creams and ointments. Tubes made of tin are used to package certain sterile formulations. Typically, the formulation is aseptically filled into the pre-sterilized tubes. However, the most common metal tubes in current use are made of aluminium with an internal lacquered surface. With this package, the tube remains collapsed as the product is removed. These tubes are frequently sealed at both ends and the nozzle must be punctured to access the product. An alternative seal that can be used with these packages is a heat seal band between the closure and the container. This band must be torn to gain access to the container contents.

Plastic tubes made from a variety of materials are superseding metal tubes. For example, the tube sleeve may be made of LDPE with either a LDPE or HDPE head or the entire tube may be made of polypropylene.

Unit-dose packaging

This term usually means that a single item such as a tablet or capsule or a specific dose is enclosed within its own disposable packaging. The most commonly used methods for unit-dose packaging are blister packs and strip packs.

Blister packs

These are used for packaging unit doses of tablets and capsules and can act as an aid for patient compliance. The medication is placed in a compartment in a base material made of paper, board, plastic or metal foil or a combination of these. The blister is generally composed of a thermoformed plastic sheet such as PVC. The protection given by the plastic blister depends on its composition, design and the method used to form it. Perforations in the base material allow individual sections of the package to be broken off. Blister packages are rigid, unlike strip packs, which are flexible.

Strip packaging

With strip packaging, two webs of material sandwich various types of medicine such as tablets, capsules, suppositories or pessaries. Each of these dosage forms is contained within its own compartment. The composition of the two webs can be selected to meet the necessary protective requirements for the medicine. Aluminium foil is commonly used to manufacture strip packs and provides a good barrier against moisture penetration. The foil is used as a laminate in which the other components add strength to the fragile aluminium foil. They also block small holes, which can occur in the thinner foil layer.

Paper

Paper is used more than any other material in packaging. Although it has an insignificant role in primary packaging, it remains the predominant secondary and tertiary packaging material. In this role, it is used as the carton which contains the primary package and, in the form of board, is the corrugated shipping container which contains both.

Patient pack dispensing

A patient pack consists of a course of medication, together with a patient information leaflet in a ready to dispense pack. Liquid formulations are supplied in a standard pack. Solid dose forms are supplied as a strip or blister pack. The size of the sealed patient pack is based on a 28, 30 or 56 dose unit appropriate to the medicine. It is supplied in this amount unless a doctor prescribes that a different quantity of medicine is to be dispensed. The patient pack is designed as a balance between the need for child resistance and the need for ease of opening. If requested by the patient, the pack contents can be repackaged in a more suitable container.

Advantages of patient packs

- They contain product information such as product and manufacturer identification and the batch number
- More efficient dispensing results in greater opportunity for patient counselling
- More information is supplied to the patient about the product.

Disadvantages of patient packs

- Increased storage space is required
- Elderly and debilitated patients may experience difficulty in opening the pack.

Key points

- Containers should preserve the quality of a medicine for its stated shelf-life
- Glass has both advantages and disadvantages in use, but remains the preferred material in many situations
- The types of glass have different uses
- Plastics may be thermosets or thermoplastics
- A variety of additives to plastics may enter medicines with which they are in contact
- CRCs may have alignment closures (Snap-safe) or push and turn (Clic-loc)
- Use of CRCs is a professional requirement for dispensed medicines unless requested otherwise
- Tamper-evident closures indicate that there has been no unlawful access to the medicine
- Aluminium is being replaced by plastics for collapsible tubes
- Unit dosage packaging may be either blister or strip packaging
- The main use for paper is for cartons and boxes
- A patient pack consists of the medicine and patient information leaflet in a ready to dispense outer pack

Chapter | 5 |

Solutions

Arthur J. Winfield

STUDY POINTS

- Definitions of solutions and expressions of solubility
- Advantages and disadvantages of using solutions
- Methods of controlling solubility
- Selection of vehicles
- Use of preservatives and other ingredients in solutions
- Principles of dispensing
- Solutions for oral use
- Diluents
- Mouthwashes
- Nasal, oral and aural solutions
- Enemas
- Use of oral syringes

Introduction

Solutions are homogeneous mixtures of two or more components. They contain one or more solutes dissolved in one or more solvents, usually solids dissolved in liquids. The solvent is often aqueous but can be oily, alcoholic or some other solvent.

There are many types of pharmaceutical solutions. Solutions may be used as oral dosage forms, mouthwashes, gargles, nasal drops and ear drops and externally as lotions, liniments, paints, etc. Solutions may also be used in injections and ophthalmic preparations (see Chs 12 and 13).

Solutions for oral dosage

Oral solutions are usually formulated so that the patient receives the usual dose of the medication in a conveniently administered volume, 5 mL or a multiple thereof, given to the patient using a 5 mL medicine spoon.

Advantages of solutions for oral use over a solid dosage form are that liquids are much easier to swallow than tablets or capsules and the medicament is readily absorbed from the gastrointestinal tract. Ease of taking is especially useful for children, elderly patients or those with chronic conditions, such as Parkinson's disease, who may have difficulty swallowing a solid oral dosage form. An advantage of solutions over suspensions is that the medicament is dispersed homogeneously throughout the preparation, without the need to shake the bottle. This makes the preparation easier for the patient to use and should ensure consistent dosage. Sometimes substances with a low aqueous solubility may be made into solution by the addition of another solvent rather than formulate the medicine as a suspension.

Disadvantages of solutions are that they are bulky, not convenient to carry around and less microbiologically and chemically stable than their solid counterparts. Oral solutions may have an unpleasant taste. The accuracy of oral dosage is dependent on the patient measuring the dose carefully.

The different forms of oral solutions are:

- *Syrups*, which are aqueous solutions that contain sugar. An example is Epilim syrup (sodium valproate)
- *Elixirs*, which are clear, flavoured liquids containing a high proportion of sucrose or a suitable polyhydric alcohol and sometimes ethanol. Examples are phenobarbital elixir and chloral elixir (see Example 5.5)
- *Linctuses*, which are viscous liquids used in the treatment of cough. They usually contain a high proportion of sucrose, other sugars or a suitable polyhydric alcohol or alcohols. Examples are Simple Linctus BP and diamorphine linctus (see Example 5.4)
- *Mixtures* is a term often used to describe pharmaceutical oral solutions and suspensions. Examples are chloral hydrate mixture and ammonium and Ipecacuanha mixture BP (see Example 5.3)

- *Oral drops* are oral solutions or suspensions which are administered in small volumes, using a suitable measuring device. A proprietary example is Abidec vitamin drops.

Containers for dispensed solutions for oral use

Plain, amber medicine bottles should be used, with a reclosable child-resistant closure. Exceptions to this are: if the medicine is in an original pack or patient pack, if there are no suitable child-resistant containers for a particular liquid preparation or if the patient requests it, e.g. if they have severe arthritis in their hands. Advice to store away from children should then be given. A 5-mL medicine spoon or an appropriate oral syringe should be supplied to the patient.

Special labels and advice for dispensed oral solutions

An expiry date should appear on the label for extemporaneously prepared solutions. Most 'official' mixtures and some oral solutions are freshly or recently prepared. 'Official' elixirs and linctuses and manufactured products are generally more stable, unless diluted. Diluted products generally have a shorter shelf-life than the undiluted preparation. Linctuses should be sipped and swallowed slowly, without the addition of water.

Solutions for other pharmaceutical uses

Topical solutions for external use are considered in Chapter 8. Some topical solutions are designed for use in body cavities, such as the nose, mouth and ear.

Mouthwashes and gargles

Gargles are used to relieve or treat sore throats and mouthwashes are used on the mucous membranes of the oral cavity, rather than the throat, to refresh and mechanically clean the mouth. Both are concentrated solutions, although gargles tend to contain higher concentrations of active ingredients than mouthwashes. Both are usually diluted with warm water before use. They may contain antiseptics, analgesics or weak astringents. The liquid is usually not intended for swallowing. Examples are Phenol Gargle BPC and Compound Sodium Chloride Mouthwash BP (see Example 5.7). Proprietary examples are chlorhexidine (Corsodyl) mouthwash and povidone-iodine (Betadine) mouthwash.

Containers for mouthwashes and gargles

An amber medicine bottle should be used for these extemporaneously prepared solutions.

Special labels and advice for mouthwashes and gargles

Directions for diluting the preparations should be given to the patient. If the preparation is not intended for swallowing, the following label is appropriate: 'Not to be swallowed in large amounts'.

Nasal solutions

Most nasal preparations are solutions, administered as nose drops or sprays. They are usually formulated to be isotonic to nasal secretions (equivalent to 0.9% normal saline) and buffered to the normal pH range of nasal fluids (pH5.5–6.5) to prevent damage to ciliary transport in the nose. The most frequent use of nose drops is as a decongestant for the common cold or to administer local steroids for the treatment of allergic rhinitis. Examples are normal saline nose drops and ephedrine nose drops, 0.5% or 1%. Overuse of topical decongestants can lead to oedema of the nasal mucosa and they should only be used for short periods of time (about 4 days) to avoid rebound congestion, called rhinitis medicamentosa. The nasal route may also be useful for new biologically active peptides and polypeptides which need to avoid the first pass metabolism and destruction by the gastrointestinal fluids. The nasal mucosa rapidly absorbs applied medicaments to give a systemic effect. There are some products utilizing nasal delivery currently available on the market, e.g. desmopressin (e.g. Desmospray, DDAVP), used in the treatment of pituitary diabetes insipidus. Accurate dosage is achieved using metered spray devices.

Ear drops

Ear drops are solutions of one or more active ingredient which exert a local effect in the ear, e.g. by softening earwax or treating infection or inflammation. They may also be referred to as *otic* or *aural preparations*. Propylene glycol, oils, glycerol (to increase viscosity) and water may be used as vehicles. Examples are aluminium acetate ear drops, almond oil ear drops and Sodium Bicarbonate Ear Drops BP (see Example 5.8).

Containers for nasal and aural preparations

Nose and ear drops that are prepared extemporaneously should be packed in an amber, ribbed hexagonal glass bottle which is fitted with a teat and dropper. Manufactured nasal solutions may be packed in flexible plastic bottles which deliver a fine spray to the nose when squeezed, or in a plain glass bottle with a pump spray or dropper. Manufactured ear drops are usually packed in small glass or plastic containers with a dropper.

Special labels and advice for nasal and aural preparations

Patients should be advised not to share nasal sprays or nose and ear drops in order to minimize contamination and infection. Manufactured nasal sprays and nose and ear drops will usually contain instructions for administration. Patients should be given advice on how to administer extemporaneously prepared nose and ear drops, accompanied by written information if possible (Fig. 5.1). For nose drops, it may be easier if the patient is lying flat with the head tilted back as far as comfortable, preferably over the edge of a bed. The patient should remain in this position for a few minutes after the drops have been administered to allow the medication to spread in the nose.

For ear drops, it may be easier for someone other than the patient to administer the drops. If desired, the drops can be warmed by holding the bottle in the hands before putting them in, but they must not be overheated. The ear lobe should be held up and back in adults, down and back in children, to allow the medication to run in deeper.

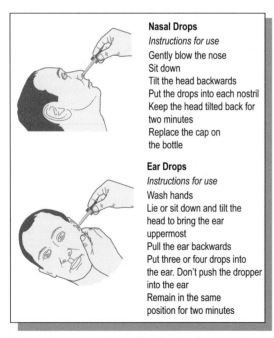

Nasal Drops
Instructions for use
Gently blow the nose
Sit down
Tilt the head backwards
Put the drops into each nostril
Keep the head tilted back for two minutes
Replace the cap on the bottle

Ear Drops
Instructions for use
Wash hands
Lie or sit down and tilt the head to bring the ear uppermost
Pull the ear backwards
Put three or four drops into the ear. Don't push the dropper into the ear
Remain in the same position for two minutes

Fig. 5.1 Patient instruction leaflets for use of nose and ear drops.

They may cause some transient stinging. If the drops are intended to soften earwax, then the ears should be syringed after several days of use.

Extemporaneous preparations should be labelled with the appropriate expiry date following the official monographs. 'For external use' is not an appropriate label and so 'Not to be taken' is advised.

Enemas

Enemas are oily or aqueous solutions that are administered rectally. They are usually anti-inflammatory, purgative, sedative or given to allow X-ray examination of the lower bowel. Examples are arachis oil enema and magnesium sulphate enema. Retention enemas are administered to give either a local action of the drug, e.g. prednisolone, or for systemic absorption, e.g. diazepam. They are used after defecation. The patient lies on one side during administration and remains there for 30 minutes to allow distribution of the medicament. Micro-enemas are single-dose, small-volume solutions. Examples are solutions of sodium phosphate, sodium citrate or docusate sodium. They are packaged in plastic containers with a nozzle for insertion into the rectum. Large-volume (0.5–1 L) enemas should be warmed to body temperature before administration.

Enemas are packed in amber glass bottles. Manufactured enemas will usually be packed in disposable polythene or polyvinyl chloride bags sealed to a rectal nozzle.

Special labels and advice for enemas

Patients should be advised on how to use the enema if they are self-administering and the time that the product will take to work. The label 'For rectal use only' should be used.

Expression of concentration

Strengths of pharmaceutical solutions can be expressed in a number of ways. The two most commonly used are in terms of amount of drug contained in 5 mL of vehicle or percentage strength (see Ch. 1).

Formulation of solutions

Solutions comprise the medicinal agent in a solvent as well as any additional agents. These additional agents are usually included to provide colour, flavour, sweetness or stability to the formulation. Most solutions are now manufactured on a large scale although it may be occasionally required to make up a solution extemporaneously. When compounding a solution, information on solubility and stability of each of the solutes must be taken into account.

Chemical and physical interactions that may take place between constituents must also be taken into account, as these will affect the preparation's stability or potency. For example, esters of *p*-hydroxybenzoic acid, which can be used as preservatives in oral solutions, have a tendency to partition into certain flavouring oils. This could reduce the effective concentration of the preservative agent in the aqueous vehicle of the preparation to a level lower than that required for preservative action.

Solubility

The saturation solubility of a chemical in a solvent is the maximum concentration of a solution, which may be prepared at a given temperature. For convenience, this is usually simply called *solubility*. Solubilities for medicinal agents in a given solvent are given in the *British Pharmacopoeia* (BP) and *Martindale* and other reference sources. Solubilities are usually stated as the number of parts of solvent (by volume) that will dissolve one part (by weight or volume) of the substance. In other situations, words are used to describe the solubility (see Examples 5.1 and 5.2). Using this information, it is often possible to calculate whether a solution can be prepared. Most solutions for pharmaceutical use are not saturated with solute.

Example 5.1

Potassium chloride is soluble in 2.8–3 parts of water.
This means that 1 g of potassium chloride will dissolve in 2.8–3 mL of water at a temperature of 20°C (taken as normal room temperature).

Example 5.2

Diazepam is described as being 'very slightly soluble' in water (which means 1 in 1000 to 1 in 10,000), 'soluble' in alcohol (which means 1 in 10 to 1 in 30) and 'freely soluble' in chloroform (which means 1 in 1 to 1 in 10).
This means that 1 g of diazepam will dissolve in between 10 and 30 mL of alcohol, but would need 1000–10,000 mL of water to dissolve, at a temperature of 20°C.

Vehicles

In pharmacy, the medium which contains the ingredients of a medicine is called the *vehicle*. In solutions, this is the solvent. The choice of a vehicle depends on the intended use of the preparation and on the nature and physicochemical properties of the active ingredients.

Water as a vehicle

Water is the vehicle used for most pharmaceutical preparations. It is widely available, relatively inexpensive, palatable and non-toxic for oral use and non-irritant for external use. It is also a good solvent for many ionizable drugs. Different types of water are available as outlined below:

- *Potable water* is drinking water, drawn freshly from a mains supply. It should be palatable and safe for drinking. Its chemical composition may include mineral impurities, which could react with drugs, e.g. the presence of calcium carbonate in hard water
- *Purified water* is prepared from suitable potable water by distillation, by treatment with ion-exchange materials or by any other suitable treatment method such as reverse osmosis. Distilled water is purified water that has been prepared by distillation
- *Water for preparations* is potable or freshly boiled and cooled purified water, which can be used in oral or external preparations which are not intended to be sterile. The boiling removes dissolved oxygen and carbon dioxide from solution in the water. Any stored water, for example drawn from a local storage tank, should not be used because of the risk of contamination with microorganisms
- *Water for injections* is pyrogen-free distilled water, sterilized immediately after collection and used for parenteral products (for further details, see Ch. 12).
- *Aromatic waters* are near-saturated aqueous solutions of volatile oils or other aromatic or volatile substances, and are often used as a vehicle in oral solutions. Some have a mild carminative action, e.g. dill. Aromatic waters are usually prepared from a concentrated ethanolic solution, in a dilution of 1 part of concentrated water with 39 parts of water. Chloroform water is used as an antimicrobial preservative and also adds sweetness to preparations.

Other vehicles used in pharmaceutical solutions

- *Syrup BP* is a solution of 66.7% sucrose in water. It will promote dental decay and is unsuitable for diabetic patients. Hydrogenated glucose syrup, mannitol, sorbitol, xylitol, etc. can replace the sucrose to give 'sugar-free' solvents

- *Alcohol (ethyl alcohol, ethanol).* This is rarely used for internal preparations but is a useful solvent for external preparations
- *Glycerol (glycerin)* may be used alone as a vehicle in some external preparations. It is viscous and miscible both with water and alcohol. It may be added as a stabilizer and sweetener in internal preparations. In concentrations above 20% v/v, it acts as a preservative
- *Propylene glycol* is a less viscous liquid and a better solvent than glycerol
- *Oils.* Bland oils such as fractionated coconut oil and arachis oil may be used for fat-soluble compounds, e.g. Calciferol Oral Solution BP. Care is required when using nut oils due to hypersensitivity reactions
- *Acetone* is used as a co-solvent in external preparations
- *Solvent ether* can be used as a co-solvent in external preparations for preoperative skin preparation. The extreme volatility of ether and risk of fire and explosion limit its usefulness.

Factors affecting solubility

Compounds that are predominantly non-polar tend to be more soluble in non-polar solvents, such as chloroform or a vegetable oil. Polar compounds tend to be more soluble in polar solvents, such as water and ethanol. The pH will also affect solubility, as many drugs are weak acids or bases. The ionized form of a compound will be the most water soluble, therefore a weakly basic drug will be most soluble in an aqueous solution that is acidic. Acid or alkali may therefore be added to manipulate solubility. Most compounds are more soluble at higher temperatures. Particle size reduction will increase the rate of solution.

Increasing the solution of compounds with low solubility

Co-solvency

The addition of co-solvents, such as ethanol, glycerol, propylene glycol or sorbitol, can increase the solubility of weak electrolytes and non-polar molecules in water.

Solubilization

Surfactants may be used as solubilizing agents. Above the critical micelle concentration (CMC), they form micelles which are used to help dissolve poorly soluble compounds. The dissolved compound may be in the centre of the micelle, adsorbed onto the micelle surface, or sit at some intermediate point, depending on the polarity of the compound. Examples of surfactants used in oral solutions are polysorbates, while soaps are used to solubilize phenolic disinfectants for external use.

Preservation of solutions

Most water-containing pharmaceutical solutions will support microbial growth unless this is prevented. Contamination may come from raw materials or be introduced during extemporaneous dispensing.

Preservatives may be added to the formulation to reduce or prevent microbial growth. Chloroform is the most widely used in oral extemporaneous preparations, although there are disadvantages to its use, including its high volatility and reported carcinogenicity in animals. Use in the UK is limited to a chloroform content of 0.5% (w/w or w/v). For oral solutions, chloroform at a strength of 0.25% v/v will usually be incorporated as Chloroform Water BP. Alternatively, double strength chloroform water may be included in pharmaceutical formulae as half the total volume of the solution, to effectively give single strength chloroform water in the finished medicine (see Example 5.3). Benzoic acid at a strength of 0.1% w/v is also suitable for oral administration, as are ethanol, sorbic acid, the hydroxybenzoate esters and syrup. Some of the alternative preservatives have pH-dependent activity.

Syrups can be preserved by the maintenance of a high concentration of sucrose as part of the formulation. Concentrations of sucrose greater than 65% w/w will usually protect an oral liquid from growth of most microorganisms by its osmotic effects. A problem with their use occurs when other ingredients are added to the syrup, as this dilutes the syrup. This may cause a loss in the preservative action of the sucrose. Accidental dilution by, for example, using a damp bottle, may have a similar effect.

Preservatives used in external solutions include chlorocresol (0.1% w/v), chlorbutanol (0.5% w/v) and the para-hydroxybenzoates (parabens).

Additional ingredients

Solutions that are intended for oral use may contain excipients such as flavouring, sweetening and, sometimes, colouring agents. These are added to improve the palatability and appearance of a solution for the patient. Stabilizing and viscosity enhancing agents may also be used.

Flavouring agents

Flavours added to solutions can make a medicine more acceptable to take, especially if the drug has an unpleasant taste. Selection of flavours is a complex process in the pharmaceutical industry. Flavours should be chosen to mask particular taste types, e.g. a fruit flavour helps to disguise an acid taste. The age of the patient should be taken into account when selecting a flavour, as children will tend to enjoy fruit or sweet flavours. Some flavours are associated with particular uses, e.g. peppermint is associated with antacid preparations. The flavour and colour should also complement each other. Extemporaneous medicines tend to use natural flavours added as juices (raspberry), extracts (liquorice), spirits (lemon and orange), syrups (blackcurrant), tinctures (ginger) and aromatic waters (anise and cinnamon). Some synthetic flavours are used in manufactured medicines.

Sweetening agents

Many oral solutions are sweetened with sugars, including glucose and sucrose. Sucrose enhances the viscosity of liquids and also gives a pleasant texture in the mouth. Prolonged use of liquid medicines containing sugar will lead to an increased incidence of dental caries, particularly in children. Attempts should be made to formulate oral solutions without sugar as a sweetening agent, using sorbitol, mannitol, xylitol, saccharin and aspartame as alternatives. Oral liquid preparations that do not contain fructose, glucose or sucrose are labelled 'sugar free' in the *British National Formulary* (BNF). These alternatives should be used where possible.

Colouring agents

Colouring agents are added to pharmaceutical preparations to enhance the appearance of a preparation or to increase the acceptability of a preparation to the patient. Colours are often matched to the flavour of a preparation, e.g. a yellow colour for a banana-flavoured preparation. Colour is also useful to give a consistent appearance where there is natural variation between batches. Colours can give distinctive appearances to some medicines, e.g. the green colour of the *Drug Tariff* formula of methadone mixture.

Colouring agents should be non-toxic and free of any therapeutic activity themselves. Natural colourants are most likely to meet this criterion and include materials derived from plants and animals, e.g. carotenoids, chlorophylls, saffron, red beetroot extract, caramel and cochineal. As with all natural agents, the disadvantage is that batches may vary in quality. Synthetic organic dyes such as the azo compounds are alternatives for colouring pharmaceutical solutions as they give a wide range of bright, stable colours. Colours appear in pharmaceutical formulae less often now, especially in children's medicines. Some consumers see their use as unnecessary and some colouring agents, e.g. tartrazine, have been implicated in allergic reactions and hyperactivity of children. Additionally, coloured dyes in medicines can lead to confusion when diagnosing diseases, e.g. a red dye appearing in vomit could be wrongly assumed to be blood. In the European Union, colours are selected from a list permitted for medicinal products, with designated 'E' numbers between 100 and 180.

Stabilizers

Antioxidants may be used where ingredients are liable to degradation by oxidation, e.g. in oils. Those which are added to oral preparations include ascorbic acid, citric acid, sodium metabisulphite and sodium sulphite. These are odourless, tasteless and non-toxic.

Viscosity-enhancing agents

Syrups may be added to increase the viscosity of an oral liquid. They also improve palatability and ease pourability. Other thickening agents may also be used (see Ch. 6).

Shelf-life of solutions

There may be individual variations, but most solutions which are prepared extemporaneously should be freshly or recently prepared. The data sheets should be consulted for information about particular manufactured solutions and for storage conditions.

Oral syringes

If fractional doses are prescribed for oral liquids, they should not be diluted, but an oral syringe should be supplied with the dispensed oral liquid. The standard 5 mL or 10 mL capacity oral syringe is marked in 0.2 mL divisions to measure fractional doses. An adapter fits into the neck of all common sizes of the medicine bottle. Instructions should be supplied with the oral syringe: 'Shake the bottle and then remove the lid and insert the adapter firmly into the top of the bottle. Push the tip of the oral syringe into the hole in the adapter and turn the bottle upside down. Pull the syringe plunger to draw liquid to the appropriate volume. It may be desirable to indicate this on the syringe. Turn the bottle right way up and carefully remove the syringe, holding the barrel. Gently put the tip into the child's mouth to be inside the cheek. Slowly and gently push the plunger in and allow the child to swallow the medicine before removing the syringe. Do not squirt the liquid or direct it towards the throat. After completing the process, remove the adapter and replace the cap on the bottle. The adapter and syringe should be rinsed and left to dry'. Patient information leaflets are available to accompany the oral syringe.

Diluents

If a prescriber insists that a manufactured solution is diluted, then a suitable diluent must be selected. Information sources to obtain this information are the *Medicines Compendium* or the National Pharmaceutical Association (NPA) *Diluent Directory*. An indication of the expiry date for the diluted preparation is also given in these references. The dilution should be freshly prepared.

A short shelf-life for a diluted solution may require patients to return to the pharmacy to collect the balance of their medication. This may happen, for instance, where an oral sodium chloride solution has been prescribed for 1 month. The solution has a 2-week expiry, and must therefore be supplied in two instalments. The patient, or their representative, should be issued with an owing slip, or some similar documentation. This should state the name of the patient, the pharmacy, the item and quantity of medicine owed and the date of issue. A record should also be kept in the pharmacy. Most computer labelling systems have the facility to handle 'owings'.

Example 5.3 **Prepare 100 mL of Ammonium and Ipecacuanha Mixture BP.**

	Master formula	For 100 mL
Ammonium bicarbonate	200 mg	2 g
Liquorice liquid extract	0.5 mL	5 mL
Ipecacuanha tincture	0.3 mL	3 mL
Concentrated camphor water	0.1 mL	1 mL
Concentrated anise water	0.05 mL	0.5mL
Double strength chloroform water	5 mL	50 mL
Water	to 10 mL	to 100 mL

Traditionally used as an expectorant cough preparation but no longer recommended.

Formulation notes. Ammonium bicarbonate, ipecacuanha and camphor water are mild expectorants. Anise water acts as a mild expectorant and a flavouring agent. Liquid liquorice extract is used as a mild expectorant, flavouring and sweetening agent. Chloroform water acts as a sweetener and a preservative. Ammonium bicarbonate is soluble 1 in 5 of water, so will dissolve to give a solution. All other ingredients are liquids.

Method of preparation. Weigh the ammonium bicarbonate on

a suitable balance and dissolve in approximately 15 mL of water, in a 100 mL conical measure. Add the double strength chloroform water to this solution. Measure the other liquid ingredients and add to the solution. Make up to volume with water in the conical measure. Pack into an amber medicine bottle with a child-resistant closure. Polish the bottle and label, and provide a 5-mL spoon.

Shelf-life and storage. Store in a cool, dry place. It is recently prepared, therefore a shelf-life of 2–3 weeks is applicable.

Advice and labelling. 'Shake well before use'. While this is not strictly required, it is good practice to include it.

Example 5.4 **Prepare 200 mL of Diamorphine Linctus.**

	Master formula	For 200 mL
Diamorphine hydrochloride	3 mg	120 mg
Oxymel	1.25 mL	50 mL
Glycerol	1.25 mL	50 mL
Compound tartrazine solution	0.06 mL	2.4 mL
Syrup	to 5 mL	to 200 mL

Traditionally used as a cough suppressant in terminal care, no longer recommended.

Formulation notes. Oxymel is a solution of acetic acid, water and purified honey, used as a demulcent and sweetening agent in linctuses. Glycerol is also a demulcent and sweetener. Compound tartrazine solution is a colouring agent and syrup is a demulcent vehicle. Diamorphine is soluble 1 in 1.6 of water and 1 in 12 of alcohol, so a solution will be produced.

Method of preparation. Weigh 120 mg diamorphine on an appropriate balance. Transfer to a 200-mL measuring cylinder. Dissolve the diamorphine in the oxymel and glycerol. Add about 50 mL of syrup, then add the compound tartrazine solution. Transfer to a previously tared amber medicine bottle (see Ch. 4). Make up to volume with the syrup in the tared bottle in order to overcome difficulties in draining all the viscous mixture from a measure. Close with a child-resistant closure, polish and label the bottle and give a 5-mL medicine spoon or oral syringe with the medicine (depending on the dosage prescribed).

Shelf-life and storage. Store in a cool, dry place. It is recently prepared, therefore a shelf-life of 2–3 weeks is applicable.

Advice and labelling. 'Shake well before use'. The linctus should be sipped and swallowed slowly, undiluted.

'Warning. This medicine may make you sleepy. If this happens, do not drive or use tools or machines. Do not drink alcohol' (BNF Label 2). Since this patient is terminally ill, they are unlikely to be driving or operating machinery so this part of the advisory label can be omitted. Alcohol should be avoided, as this will increase the sedative effect.

Example 5.5 **Prepare 50 mL of Chloral Elixir, Paediatric.**

	Master formula	For 50 mL
Chloral hydrate	200 mg	2 g
Water	0.1 mL	1 mL
Blackcurrant syrup	1 mL	10 mL
Syrup	to 5 mL	to 50 mL

Action and uses. Traditionally used for short-term use in insomnia.

Formulation notes. Chloral hydrate is soluble 1 in 0.3 of water and has an unpleasant taste. Blackcurrant syrup is used as a flavouring agent to mask this.

Method of preparation. Weigh 2 g chloral hydrate on a suitable balance. Transfer it to a 50-mL measuring cylinder and dissolve it in water. Add the blackcurrant syrup. Add some of the syrup (rinsing the measure used for the blackcurrant syrup). Transfer the mixture to a tared, 50-mL amber medicine bottle and make up to volume, to avoid loss of the viscous product in the measures. Polish and label the bottle and give a 5-mL medicine spoon or oral syringe with the medicine.

Shelf-life and storage. Store in a cool, dry place. Chloral hydrate is volatile and sensitive to light. It is recently prepared and a shelf life of 2–3 weeks is appropriate.

Advice and labelling. 'Shake well before use' and BNF Labels 1 and 27. An appropriate dose for a child up to 1 year is one 5-mL spoonful to be given, well diluted with wa-

Example 5.6 **Prepare 200 mL of Potassium Citrate Mixture BP.**

	Master formula	For 200 mL
Potassium citrate	3 g	60 g
Citric acid monohydrate	500 mg	10 g
Syrup	2.5 mL	50 mL
Quillaia tincture	0.1 mL	2 mL

Lemon spirit	0.05 mL	1 mL
Double strength chloroform water	3 mL	60 mL
Water	to 10 mL	to 200 mL

ter, at bedtime. The parent should be advised that this might make the child drowsy.

Traditionally used for the alkalinization of urine to relieve discomfort in mild urinary tract infections or cystitis.

Formulation notes. Citric acid and potassium citrate are the active ingredients; both are soluble 1 in 1 of water. Lemon spirit, which is lemon oil in alcoholic solution, is a flavouring agent. The oil tends to be displaced from solution in an aqueous medium, especially in the presence of a high concentration of salts. The quillaia tincture is a surfactant used to emulsify any displaced lemon oil. Syrup is a sweetening agent.

Method of preparation. The solids should be size reduced, weighed and dissolved in the double strength chloroform water and syrup. The quillaia tincture should be added before the lemon spirit is added with stirring, so that immediate emulsification of the oil will be achieved if required. Make up to volume with water. Pack in an amber medicine bottle with a child-resistant closure. Polish and label the bottle and give a 5-mL medicine spoon with the medicine.

Shelf-life and storage. Store in a cool, dry place. It is recently prepared, therefore a shelf-life of 2–3 weeks is applicable.

Advice and labelling. 'Shake well before use'. The medicine should be diluted with plenty of water (BNF Label 27).

Example 5.7 **Prepare 500 mL of Compound Sodium Chloride Mouthwash BP.**

	Master formula	For 500 mL
Sodium chloride	1.5 g	7.5 g
Sodium bicarbonate	1 g	5 g
Concentrated peppermint emulsion	2.5 mL	12.5 mL
Double strength chloroform water	50 mL	250 mL
Water	to 100 mL	to 500 mL

Action and uses. Mechanically cleans and freshens the mouth.

Formulation notes. Concentrated peppermint emulsion is used as a flavouring and the chloroform water is a sweetener and preservative. Sodium chloride is soluble 1 in 3 of water and sodium bicarbonate is soluble 1 in 11 of water.

Method of preparation. The solids are weighed on a suitable balance and dissolved in a 500-mL conical measure in approximately 100 mL of water. Add the double strength chloroform water and the concentrated peppermint emulsion. Make up to volume with water. Pack in an amber bottle with a child-resistant closure. Polish and label the bottle.

Shelf-life and storage. Store in a cool, dry place. It is recently prepared, therefore a shelf-life of 2–3 weeks is applicable.

Advice and labelling. 'Shake well before use'. The patient should be directed to use about 15 mL diluted in an equal volume of warm water, usually morning and night, unless otherwise directed. The solution should be used as a mouthwash and should not be swallowed, although reassure the patient that it is not harmful to swallow small amounts of the mouthwash.

Example 5.8 **Prepare 10 mL of Sodium Bicarbonate Ear Drops BP.**

	Master formula	For 10 mL
Sodium bicarbonate	5 g	500 mg
Glycerol	30 mL	3 mL
Water	to 100 mL	to 10 mL

Action and uses. For the softening and removal of earwax (usually before syringing with warm water).

Formulation notes. Sodium bicarbonate is soluble 1 in 11 of water. Glycerol is a viscous liquid used to thicken the drops, but presents problems in measuring the volume accurately.

Method of preparation. Weigh 500 mg sodium bicarbonate and dissolve in 6 mL of water, using a 10-mL conical measure. Carefully make up to 7 mL using water. Carefully add glycerol up to the 10-mL mark (this will result in 3 mL of glycerol being added to the solution). Pack in a 10-mL hexagonal, amber, ribbed bottle with a dropper. Polish and label the bottle on the three smooth sides.

Shelf-life and storage. Store in a cool, dry place. The drops are recently prepared, therefore a shelf-life of 2–3 weeks is applicable.

Advice and labelling. 'Shake well before use' and 'Not to be taken'. The bottle may be warmed in the hands before placing drops in the ears. A patient information leaflet should be used to describe how to use the drops (see Fig. 5.1).

Key points

- Pharmaceutical solutions are given different names depending on their nature and use
- There are both advantages and disadvantages in the use of oral solutions
- Solutions may also be used for mouthwashes, gargles, nasal drops and sprays, ear drops and enemas
- Many different vehicles may be used in pharmaceutical solutions, but water is the most common
- Saturation solubility of a drug in a solvent is affected by polarity of both drug and solvent
- Saturation solubility can be increased by techniques such as co-solvency and solubilization
- Antimicrobial preservation is required for most aqueous solutions
- Various additives such as flavours, sweeteners and colours may be added to improve the palatability of oral solutions
- Oral syringes will be required for doses of less than 5 mL and its use explained

Chapter 6

Suspensions

Arthur J. Winfield

STUDY POINTS

- The nature of suspensions
- The pharmaceutical uses of suspensions
- The properties of an ideal suspension
- Formulating a suspension
- Ingredients which may be added to suspensions
- The dispensing of suspensions for internal and external use

Introduction

Suspensions contain one or more insoluble medicaments in a vehicle, with other additives such as preservatives, flavours, colours, buffers and stabilizers. Most pharmaceutical suspensions are aqueous, but an oily vehicle is sometimes used. Suspensions may be used for oral administration, inhalation, topical application, as ophthalmic preparations, for parenteral administration and as aerosols.

A pharmaceutical suspension may be defined as a disperse system in which one substance (the disperse phase) is distributed in particulate form throughout another (the continuous phase). Most are classified as a coarse suspension, which is a dispersion of particles with a mean diameter >1 μm. A colloidal suspension is a dispersion of particles with a mean diameter <1 μm. Suspended solids slowly separate on standing, but redispersion may be difficult if they form a compacted sediment.

Pharmaceutical applications of suspensions

Suspensions may be used pharmaceutically for a number of reasons. Some are given below:

- Drugs with low solubility in the continuous phase can be formulated as suspensions
- Patient acceptability – a liquid form rather than a solid dosage form
- Drugs that have an unpleasant taste in their soluble form can be made into insoluble derivatives, and formulated as a suspension, which will be more palatable, e.g. chloramphenicol (soluble) and chloramphenicol palmitate (insoluble)
- In oral suspensions, the drug is delivered in finely divided form, therefore optimal dissolution occurs in the gastrointestinal (GI) fluids and hence the rate of absorption is increased
- Insoluble forms of drugs may prolong the action of a drug by preventing rapid degradation in the continuous phase
- If the drug is unstable when in contact with the vehicle, suspensions should be prepared immediately prior to handing out to the patient in order to reduce the amount of time that the drug particles are in contact with the dispersion medium. For example, in ampicillin suspension, water is added to powder or granules prior to giving out to the patient. A 14-day expiry date is given, if the product is to be kept in the fridge
- Drugs which degrade in aqueous solution may be suspended in a non-aqueous phase, e.g. tetracycline hydrochloride has been suspended in a fractionated coconut oil for ophthalmic use
- Bulky, insoluble powders can be formulated as a suspension so that they are easier to take, e.g. kaolin, chalk and magnesium trisilicate (see Examples 6.1 and 6.2)
- Intramuscular, intra-articular or subcutaneous injections are often formulated as suspensions to prolong the release of the drug
- Lotions containing insoluble solids are formulated to leave a thin coating of medicament on the skin. As the vehicle evaporates, it gives a cooling effect and leaves the solid behind. Examples are Calamine Lotion BP (see Example 6.3) and Sulphur Lotion Compound BPC (see Ch. 8).

Properties of a good pharmaceutical suspension

In preparing a pharmaceutically elegant product, several desirable properties are sought:
- There is ready redispersion of any sediment which accumulates on storage
- After gentle shaking, the medicament stays in suspension long enough for a dose to be accurately measured
- The suspension is pourable
- Particles in suspension are small and relatively uniform in size, so that the product is free from a gritty texture.

Formulation of suspensions

The three steps that can be taken to ensure formulation of an elegant pharmaceutical suspension are:
1. Control particle size. On a small scale, this can be done using a mortar and pestle, to grind down ingredients to a fine powder
2. Use a thickening agent to increase viscosity of the vehicle, by using suspending or viscosity-increasing agents
3. Use a wetting agent.

Some of the theoretical and practical aspects of these will be considered in the context of extemporaneous dispensing.

The insoluble medicament may be a diffusible solid or an indiffusible solid:

Diffusible solids (*dispersible solids*). These are insoluble solids that are light and easily wetted by water. They mix readily with water, and stay dispersed long enough for an adequate dose to be measured. After settling, they redisperse easily. Examples include magnesium trisilicate, light magnesium carbonate, bismuth carbonate and light kaolin (see Example 6.1).

Indiffusible solids. Most insoluble solids are not easily wetted, and may form large porous clumps in the liquid. These solids will not remain evenly distributed in the vehicle long enough for an adequate dose to be measured. They may not redisperse easily. Examples for internal use include phenobarbital and chalk (see Example 6.2), and for external use calamine, hydrocortisone, sulphur and zinc oxide.

Problems encountered when formulating insoluble solids into a suspension

Various factors need to be considered when formulating insoluble solids into a suspension.

Sedimentation

The factors affecting the rate of sedimentation of a particle are described in Stokes' equation:

$$v = 2gr^2 \ (\rho_1 - \rho_2)\,/9\eta$$

where v = velocity of a spherical particle of radius r, and density ρ_1, in a liquid of density ρ_2, and viscosity η, and where g is the acceleration due to gravity.

The basic consequences of this equation are that the rate of fall of a suspended particle in a vehicle of a given density is greater for larger particles than it is for smaller particles. Also, the greater the difference in density between the particles and vehicle, the greater will be the rate of descent. Increasing the viscosity of the dispersion medium, within limits, so that the suspension is still pourable, will reduce the rate of sedimentation of a solid drug. Thus a decrease in settling rate in a suspension may be achieved by reducing the size of the particles and by increasing the density and the viscosity of the continuous phase.

Flocculation

The natural tendency of particles towards aggregation will determine the properties of a suspension. In a deflocculated suspension, the dispersed solid particles remain separate and settle slowly. However, the sediment that eventually forms is hard to redisperse and is described as a 'cake' or 'clay'. In a flocculated suspension, individual particles aggregate into clumps or floccules in suspension. Because these flocs are larger than individual particles, sedimentation is more rapid, but the sediment is loose and easily redispersible. Excess flocculation may prevent 'pourability' due to its effect on rheological properties.

The ideal is to use either a deflocculated system with a sufficiently high viscosity to prevent sedimentation, or controlled flocculation with a suitable combination of rate of sedimentation, type of sediment and pourability.

Wetting

Air may be trapped in the particles of poorly wetted solids, which causes them to float to the surface of the preparation and prevents them from being readily dispersed throughout the vehicle. Wetting of the particles can be encouraged by reducing the interfacial tension between the solid and the vehicle, so that adsorbed air is displaced from solid surfaces by liquid. Suitable wetting agents have this effect, but decrease interparticular forces, thereby affecting flocculation.

Hydrophilic colloids such as acacia and tragacanth can act as wetting agents. However, care should be taken when using these agents, as they can promote deflocculation. Intermediate hydrophilic–lipophilic balance (HLB) surfactants (see Ch. 7) such as polysorbates and sorbitan esters are used for internal preparations. Solvents such as ethanol, glycerol and the glycols also facilitate wetting. Sodium lauryl sulphate and quillaia tincture are used in external preparations.

Suspending agents

Suspending agents increase the viscosity of the vehicle, thereby slowing down sedimentation. Most agents can form thixotropic gels which are semi-solid on standing, but flow readily after shaking. Care must be taken when selecting a suspending agent for oral preparations, as the acid environment of the stomach may alter the physical characteristics of the suspension, and therefore the rate of release of the drug from suspension. Some suspending agents may also bind to certain medicaments, making them less bioavailable.

Suspending agents can be divided into five broad categories: natural polysaccharides, semi-synthetic polysaccharides, clays, synthetic thickeners and miscellaneous compounds.

Natural polysaccharides

The main problem with these agents is their natural variability between batches and microbial contamination. Tragacanth is a widely used suspending agent and is less viscous at pH 4–7.5. As a rule of thumb, 0.2 g Tragacanth Powder is added per 100 mL suspension or 2 g Compound Tragacanth Powder per 100 mL suspension. Tragacanth Powder requires to be dispersed with the insoluble powders before water is added to prevent clumping (see Example 6.2). Compound Tragacanth Powder BP 1980 contains tragacanth, acacia, starch and sucrose and so is easier to use. Other examples include acacia gum, starch, agar, guar gum, carrageenan and sodium alginate. These materials should not be used externally as they leave a sticky feel on the skin.

Semi-synthetic polysaccharides

These are derived from the naturally occurring polysaccharide cellulose. Examples include methylcellulose (Cologel, Celacol), hydroxyethylcellulose (Natrosol 250), sodium carboxymethylcellulose (Carmellose sodium) and microcrystalline cellulose (Avicel).

Clays

These are naturally occurring inorganic materials, which are mainly hydrated silicates. Examples include bentonite and magnesium aluminium silicate (Veegum).

Synthetic thickeners

These were introduced to overcome the variable quality of natural products. Examples include carbomer (Carboxyvinyl polymer, Carbopol), colloidal silicon dioxide (Aerosil, Cab-o-sil) and polyvinyl alcohol.

Miscellaneous compounds

Gelatin is used as a suspending and viscosity-increasing agent.

Preservation of suspensions

Water is the most common source of microbial contamination. All pharmaceutical preparations that contain water are therefore susceptible to microbial growth. Also the naturally occurring additives such as acacia and tragacanth may be sources of microbes and spores. Preservative action may be diminished because of adsorption of the preservative onto solid particles of drug, or interaction with suspending agents. Useful preservatives in extemporaneous preparations include chloroform water, benzoic acid and hydroxybenzoates.

The dispensing of suspensions

The method of dispensing suspensions is the same for most, with some differences for specific ingredients.

- Crystalline and granular solids are finely powdered in the mortar. The suspending agent should then be added and mixed thoroughly in the mortar. Do not apply too much pressure, otherwise gumming or caking of the suspending agent will occur and heat of friction will make it sticky.
- Add a little of the liquid vehicle to make a paste and mix well until smooth and free of lumps. Continue with gradual additions until the mixture can be poured into a tared bottle. Further liquid is used to rinse all the powder into the bottle, where it is made up to volume.

Variations

- If wetting agents are included in the formulation, add them before forming the paste
- If syrup and/or glycerol are in the formulation, use this rather than water to form the initial paste
- If soluble solids are being used, dissolve them in the vehicle before or after making the paste
- Leave addition of volatile components, colourings or concentrated flavouring tinctures such as chloroform spirit, liquid liquorice extract and compound tartrazine solution until near the end.

Most 'official' suspensions will be prepared from the constituent ingredients. There may be some occasions where an oral solid dosage form, such as a tablet or capsule, will have to be reformulated by the pharmacist into an oral suspension, e.g. where the medicine is for a child (see Example 6.4). It is important to obtain as much information (physical, chemical and microbiological) as possible about the manufactured drug and its excipients. Typically, the tablet will be crushed or capsule contents emptied into the mortar and a suspending agent added. A paste is formed with the vehicle and then diluted to a suitable volume, with the addition of any other desired ingredients such as preservative or flavour. A short expiry of no more than 7 days should be given owing to the lack of knowledge about the stability of the formulation.

Containers for suspensions

Suspensions should be packed in amber bottles. There should be adequate air space above the liquid to allow shaking and ease of pouring.

Special labels and advice for suspensions

The most important additional label for suspensions is *'Shake well before use'*, as some sedimentation of medicament would normally be expected. Shaking the bottle will redisperse the medicament and ensure that the patient can measure an accurate dose.

'Store in a cool place'. Stability of suspensions may be adversely affected by both extremes and variations of temperature. Some suspensions, such as those made by reconstituting dry powders, may need to be stored in a refrigerator.

Extemporaneously prepared and reconstituted suspensions will have a relatively short shelf-life. They are usually required to be recently or freshly prepared, with a 1–4-week expiry date. Some official formulae state an expiry date, but many do not. The pharmacist may have to make judgements about the expiry date for a particular preparation, based on its constituents and likely storage conditions. The manufacturer's literature for reconstituted products will give recommended storage conditions.

Inhalations

Suspensions are useful formulations for inhalations. The volatile components are adsorbed onto the surface of a diffusible solid to ensure uniform dispersion throughout the liquid. When hot water is added, the oils vaporize. Where quantities are not stated, 1 g of light magnesium carbonate is used for each 2 mL of oil (such as eucalyptus oil) or 2 g of volatile solid (such as menthol). An example of a traditional inhalation is menthol and eucalyptus inhalation.

Example 6.1 Prepare 150 mL Kaolin and Morphine Mixture BP.

	Master formula	For 150 mL
Light kaolin	2 g	30 g
Sodium bicarbonate	500 mg	7.5 g
Chloroform and morphine tincture	0.4 mL	6 mL
Water	to 10 mL	to 150 mL

Traditionally used, but no longer recommended, for the treatment of acute diarrhoea.

Formulation notes. Light kaolin is a diffusible solid; therefore no suspending agent is required.

Method of preparation. Weigh the light kaolin and place in the mortar. Dissolve the sodium bicarbonate in about 100 mL of water. Gradually add this to the light kaolin in the mortar with mixing to disperse the solid. Add the chloroform and morphine tincture. Wash the mixture into a tared, amber medicine bottle and make up to volume with water.

Example 6.2 Prepare 100 mL of Chalk Mixture, Paediatric BP.

	Master formula	For 100 mL
Chalk	100 mg	2 g
Tragacanth	10 mg	200 mg
Syrup	0.5 mL	10 mL
Concentrated cinnamon water	0.02 mL	0.4 mL
Double strength chloroform water	2.5 mL	50 mL
Water	to 5 mL	to 100 mL

Traditionally used, but no longer recommended, as an antidiarrhoeal mixture for children.

Formulation notes. Chalk is practically insoluble in water and is an indiffusible solid, which requires a suspending agent. Tragacanth powder is used in this formulation. The concentrated cinnamon water is a flavouring agent and the syrup increases the viscosity as well as acting as a sweetener. Chloroform water is the preservative.

Method of preparation. The chalk and tragacanth should be weighed and lightly mixed in a mortar and pestle. Add the syrup and mix to make a paste. The double strength chloroform water should be gradually added, with mixing, followed by the concentrated cinnamon water. The mixture should be rinsed into a previously tared 100-mL amber medicine bottle and made up to volume with water. Seal the bottle and shake the suspension well.

Example 6.3 **Prepare 200 mL Calamine Lotion BP.**

	Master formula	For 200 mL
Calamine	15 g	30 g
Zinc oxide	5 g	10 g
Bentonite	3 g	6 g
Sodium citrate	500 mg	1 g
Liquefied phenol	0.5 mL	1 mL
Glycerol	5 mL	10 mL
Water	to 100 mL	to 200 mL

Action and uses. As a cooling lotion for sunburn or skin irritation and pruritus.

Formulation notes. Calamine is a coloured zinc carbonate and is practically insoluble in water, as is zinc oxide. Both are indiffusible solids. Sodium citrate is added to control the flocculation of calamine. Bentonite is a thickening agent and glycerol will thicken the product and help powder adherence to the skin. Liquefied phenol acts as a preservative and antiseptic.

Method of preparation. The dry powders should be weighed and mixed in a mortar so that the bentonite is well distributed. Add the glycerol to the powders and mix. The sodium citrate is dissolved in about 140 mL of water, and gradually added to the mixture in the mortar, so that a smooth paste is produced. Add the liquefied phenol, taking care not to splash, as it is caustic. Transfer the mixture to a tared, amber ribbed glass bottle, adding washings from the mortar, and make up to volume. Seal with a child-resistant closure.

Shelf-life and storage. Store in a cool, dry place. It is recently prepared; therefore a shelf-life of 2–3 weeks is applicable.

Advice and labelling. 'For external use only', 'Shake well before use' and 'Do not apply to broken skin'. The lotion should be applied to the affected areas when required and allowed to dry.

Example 6.4 **Prepare Spironolactone Suspension 15 mg/5 mL.**
Label: 5 mL 3 times a day. Send 100 mL. For a 4-year-old child.

	Master formula	For 100 mL
Spironolactone	q.s.[a]	300 mg
Compound orange spirit	0.2%	0.2 mL
Cologel	20%	20 mL
Water	to 100%	100 mL

[a]q.s. means sufficient.

Action and uses. A potassium-sparing diuretic used in oedema of heart failure and nephrotic syndrome.

Formulation notes. Spironolactone is practically insoluble in water. Cologel (methylcellulose) acts as the suspending agent. Compound orange spirit is a flavouring agent.

Method of preparation. Tablets may be used, and sufficient crushed in a mortar and pestle to give 300 mg spironolactone (e.g. 6 × 50 mg tablets). Alternatively, weigh the powder and transfer to a mortar and pestle. Add the Cologel and mix to a paste. Gradually add some of the water. Add the compound orange spirit. Rinse the suspension into a tared, amber medicine bottle and make up to volume with water. Shake the bottle well and seal with a child-resistant closure. Polish and label the bottle and give a 5-mL medicine spoon with the medicine.

Shelf-life and storage. It is recently prepared with a shelf-life of 4 weeks when stored in a refrigerator. Spironolactone should be protected from light.

Advice and labelling. 'Shake well before use' and 'Give one 5-mL spoonful 3 times a day'. BNF Label 21 should be used. Reinforce the storage conditions.

Key points

- Suspensions can be used to administer an insoluble solid by the oral route
- Suspensions may be used to replace tablets, to improve dissolution rate, to prolong action and to mask a bad taste
- Solids may be diffusible or indiffusible and require different dispensing techniques
- Stokes' equation can be applied when formulating a suspension to help ensure accurate dosage of the drug
- Flocculated particles settle quickly and redisperse easily, while deflocculated particles settle slowly but tend to cake
- Hydrophobic solids may require wetting agents
- Suspending agents are added to slow down the rate of settling of the solid
- Suspending agents may be natural polysaccharides, semi-synthetic polysaccharides, clays or synthetic polymers
- Some suspensions are made by adding water to reconstitute manufactured powders when stability is a problem
- 'Shake well before use' and 'Store in a cool place' should be part of the labels on a suspension
- Inhalations are suspensions of a volatile material adsorbed onto a diffusible solid

Chapter | 7 |

Emulsions

Arthur J. Winfield

STUDY POINTS

- The uses of pharmaceutical emulsions
- The different types of emulsion and their identification
- The formulation of emulsions
- Selection of emulsifying agents and other ingredients
- The dispensing processes for emulsions

Introduction

An emulsion consists of two immiscible liquids, one of which is uniformly dispersed throughout the other as fine droplets normally of diameter 0.1–100 μm. To prepare a stable emulsion, a third ingredient, an emulsifying agent, is required. Oral emulsions are stabilized oil-in-water dispersions that may contain one or more active ingredients. They are a useful way of presenting oils and fats in a palatable form. Emulsions for external use are known as *lotions*, *applications* or *liniments* if liquid, or *creams* if semi-solid in nature. Some parenteral products may also be formulated as emulsions. Most important of these is total parenteral nutrition (see Ch. 15). Pharmaceutically, the term 'emulsion', when no other qualification is used, is taken to mean an oil-in-water preparation for internal use.

Pharmaceutical applications of emulsions

Emulsions have a wide range of uses, including:
- Oral, rectal and topical administration of oils and oil-soluble drugs
- Formulation of oil- and water-soluble drugs together
- To enhance palatability of oils when given orally by disguising both taste and oiliness
- Increasing absorption of oils and oil-soluble drugs through intestinal walls
- Intramuscular injections of some water-soluble vaccines: these provide slow release and therefore a greater antibody response and longer-lasting immunity
- Total parenteral nutrition (see Ch. 15).

Examples of traditionally used emulsions for oral use are Cod-Liver Oil Emulsion (see Example 7.1), Liquid Paraffin Oral Emulsion BP (see Example 7.2). An example of emulsion for external use is Oily Calamine Lotion BP (see Example 7.3).

Emulsion types

Emulsions may be oil-in-water (o/w) emulsions, where oil is the disperse phase in a continuous phase of water, or water-in-oil (w/o) emulsions, where water is the disperse phase in a continuous phase of oil. It is also possible to form a multiple emulsion, e.g. a water droplet enclosed in an oil droplet, which is itself dispersed in water–a w/o/w emulsion. Multiple emulsions are increasingly used in manufactured pharmaceutical products and are used for delayed action drug delivery systems.

If the emulsion is for oral or intravenous administration, it will always be oil-in-water. Intramuscular injections may be water-in-oil for depot therapy. When selecting emulsion type for preparations for external use, the therapeutic use, texture and patient acceptability will be taken into account. Oil-in-water emulsions are less greasy, easily washed off the skin and more cosmetically acceptable than water-in-oil emulsions. They have an occlusive effect, which hydrates the upper layers of the skin (called an *emollient*, see Ch. 8). Water-in-oil emulsions rub in more easily.

Identification of emulsion type

There is a range of tests available to identify the emulsion type. Some of the tests that can be used are outlined below.

Miscibility test. An emulsion will only mix with a liquid that is miscible with its continuous phase. Therefore an o/w emulsion is miscible with water, a w/o emulsion with an oil.

Conductivity measurement. Systems with an aqueous continuous phase will conduct electricity, while systems with an oily continuous phase will not.

Staining test. A dry filter paper impregnated with cobalt chloride turns from blue to pink on exposure to stable o/w emulsions.

Dye test. If an oil-soluble dye is used, o/w emulsions are paler in colour than w/o emulsions. If examined microscopically, an o/w emulsion will appear as coloured globules on a colourless background while a w/o emulsion will appear as colourless globules against a coloured background.

Formulation of emulsions

An ideal emulsion has globules of disperse phase that retain their initial character, that is the mean globule size does not change and the globules remain evenly distributed. The formulation of emulsions involves the prevention of coalescence of the disperse phase (often called 'cracking') and reducing the rate of creaming.

Emulsifying agents

Emulsifying agents help the production of a stable emulsion by reducing interfacial tension and then maintaining the separation of the droplets by forming a barrier at the interface. Most emulsifying agents are surface-active agents. Emulsion type is determined mainly by the solubility of the emulsifying agent. If the emulsifying agent is more soluble in water (i.e. hydrophilic), then water will be the continuous phase and an o/w emulsion will be formed. If the emulsifying agent is more soluble in oil (i.e. lipophilic), oil will be the continuous phase and a w/o emulsion will be formed. If a substance is added which alters the solubility of the emulsifying agent, this balance may be altered and the emulsion may change type. The process is called *phase inversion*. The ideal emulsifying agent is colourless, odourless, tasteless, non-toxic, non-irritant and able to produce stable emulsions at low concentrations.

Emulsifying agents can be classed into three groups: naturally occurring, synthetic surfactants and finely divided solids.

Naturally occurring emulsifying agents

These agents come from vegetable or animal sources. Therefore the quality may vary from batch to batch and they are susceptible to microbial contamination and degradation.

Polysaccharides. Acacia is the best emulsifying agent for extemporaneously prepared oral emulsions as it forms a thick film at the oil–water interface to act as a barrier to coalescence. It is too sticky for external use. Tragacanth is used to increase the viscosity of an emulsion and prevent creaming. Other polysaccharides, such as starch, pectin and carrageenan, are used to stabilize an emulsion.

Semi-synthetic polysaccharides. Low-viscosity grades of methylcellulose (see Example 7.2) and carboxymethylcellulose will form o/w emulsions.

Sterol-containing substances. These agents act as water-in-oil emulsifying agents. Examples include beeswax, wool fat and wool alcohols (see Ch. 8).

Synthetic surfactants

These agents are classified according to their ionic characteristics as anionic, cationic, non-ionic and ampholytic. The latter are used in detergents and soaps but are not widely used in pharmacy.

Anionic surfactants. These are organic salts which, in water, have a surface-active anion. They are incompatible with some organic and inorganic cations and with large organic cations such as cetrimide. They are widely used in external preparations as o/w emulsifying agents. They must be in their ionized form to be effective and emulsions made with anionic surfactants are generally stable at more alkaline pH.

Some pharmaceutical examples of anionic surfactants include:

- Alkali metal and ammonium soaps such as sodium stearate (o/w)
- Soaps of divalent and trivalent metals such as calcium oleate (w/o) (see Example 7.3)
- Amine soaps such as triethanolamine oleate (o/w)
- Alkyl sulphates such as sodium lauryl sulphate (o/w).

Cationic surfactants. These are usually quaternary ammonium compounds which have a surface-active cation and so are sensitive to anionic surfactants and drugs. They are used in the preparation of o/w emulsions for external use and must be in their ionized form to be effective. Emulsions formed by a cationic surfactant are generally stable at acidic pH. The cationic surfactants also have antimicrobial activity. Examples include cetrimide and benzalkonium chloride.

Non-ionic surfactants. These are synthetic materials and make up the largest group of surfactants. They are used to produce either o/w or w/o emulsions for both external and internal use. The non-ionic surfactants are compatible with both anionic and cationic substances and are highly resistant to pH change. The type of emulsion formed depends on the balance between hydrophilic and lipophilic groups which is expressed as the HLB (hydrophilic–lipophilic balance) number (see below). Examples of the main types include glycol and glycerol esters, macrogol ethers and esters, sorbitan esters and polysorbates.

The HLB (hydrophilic–lipophilic balance) system. A HLB number, usually between 1 and 20, is allocated to an emulsifying agent and represents the relative proportions of the lipophilic and hydrophilic parts of the molecule. The lower the number, the more oil soluble the emulsifying agent. Higher numbers (8–18) indicate a hydrophilic molecule which produces an o/w emulsion. Low numbers (3–6) indicate a lipophilic molecule which produces a w/o emulsion. Oils and waxy materials have a 'required HLB number' which helps in the selection of appropriate emulsifying agents when formulating emulsions. Liquid paraffin, for example, has a required HLB value of 4 to obtain a w/o emulsion and 12 for an o/w emulsion. Two or more surfactants can be combined to achieve a suitable HLB value and often give better results than one surfactant alone. HLB values of some commonly used emulsifying agents are given in Table 7.1.

Finely divided solids

Finely divided solids can be adsorbed at the oil–water interface to form a coherent film that prevents coalescence of the dispersed globules. If the solid particles are preferentially wetted by oil, a w/o emulsion is formed. Conversely, if the particles are preferentially wetted by water, an o/w emulsion is formed. They form emulsions with good stability which are less prone to microbial contamination than those formed with other naturally derived agents. Examples are bentonite, aluminium magnesium silicate and colloidal

Table 7.1 HLB values of emulsifying agents

Emulsifying agent	HLB value
Acacia	8.0
Sorbitan laurate (Span 20)	8.6
Sorbitan stearate (Span 60)	4.7
Polysorbate 20 (Tween 20)	16.7
Polysorbate 80 (Tween 80)	15.0
Sodium lauryl sulphate	40.0
Sodium oleate	18.0
Tragacanth	13.2
Triethanolamine oleate	12.0

silicon dioxide. Colloidal aluminium and magnesium hydroxides are used for internal preparations. For example, liquid paraffin and magnesium hydroxide oral emulsion is stabilized by the magnesium hydroxide.

Choosing an emulsifying agent

The active ingredients that are to be emulsified and the intended use of the product will determine the choice of emulsifying agent. The natural polysaccharides (acacia) and non-ionic emulsifying agents are useful for internal emulsions because they are non-toxic and non-irritant. Quillaia can be used in low concentrations, but soap emulsions irritate the gastrointestinal tract and have a laxative effect. The taste should be bland and palatable, for example, natural polysaccharides. Polysorbates have a disagreeable taste, therefore flavouring ingredients are necessary. Only certain non-ionic emulsifying agents are suitable for parenteral use including lecithin, polysorbate 80, methylcellulose, gelatin and serum albumin. A wider range of emulsifying agents can be used externally, although the polysaccharides are normally considered too sticky.

Antioxidants

Some oils are liable to degradation by oxidation and therefore antioxidants may be added to the formulation. They should be preferentially soluble in the oily phase.

Antimicrobial preservatives

Emulsions contain water, which will support microbial growth. Microbes produce unpleasant odours, colour changes and gases. In addition, they may affect the emulsifying agent, possibly causing the breakdown of the emulsion. Other ingredients in emulsions can provide a growth medium for microbes. Examples include arachis oil which supports *Aspergillus* species and liquid paraffin which supports *Penicillium* species. Contamination may be introduced from a variety of sources including:
- Natural emulsifying agents, e.g. starch and acacia
- Water, if not properly stored
- Carelessly cleaned equipment
- Poor closures on containers.

Antimicrobial preservative agents should be free from toxic effects, odour, taste (for internal use) and colour. They should be bactericidal rather than bacteriostatic, have a rapid action and wide antibacterial spectrum over a range of temperatures and pH. Additionally, emulsion ingredients should not affect their activity and they should be resistant to attack by microorganisms. The effect of the partition coefficient is also important. Microbial growth normally occurs in the aqueous phase of an emulsion; therefore it is important that a sufficient concentration of preservative is present in the aqueous phase. A preservative with a low oil/

water partition coefficient will have a higher concentration in the aqueous phase. A combination of preservatives may give the best preservative cover for an emulsion system. The ratio of the disperse phase volume to the total volume is known as the *phase volume* or *phase volume ratio*. If, for example, a preservative is soluble in the oil and if the proportion of oil is increased, the concentration of preservative in the aqueous phase decreases. This could reduce the concentration in the aqueous phase below an effective concentration.

Some preservatives in use are listed below:

- Benzoic acid: effective at a concentration of 0.1% at a pH below 5
- Esters of parahydroxybenzoic acid such as methyl paraben (0.01–0.3%)
- Chloroform, as chloroform water (0.25% v/v)
- Chlorocresol (0.05–0.2%)
- Phenoxyethanol (0.5–1.0%)
- Benzyl alcohol (0.1–3%)
- Quaternary ammonium compounds, e.g. cetrimide, which can be used as a primary emulsifying agent but can also be used as a preservative
- Organic mercurial compounds such as phenyl mercuric nitrate and acetate (0.001–0.002%).

Colours and flavourings

Colour is rarely needed in an emulsion, as most have a white colour and thick texture. Emulsions for oral use will usually contain some flavouring agent.

Stability of emulsions

Phase inversion

This is the process in which an emulsion changes from one type to another, say o/w to w/o. The most stable range of disperse phase concentration is 30–60%. As the amount of disperse phase approaches or exceeds a theoretical maximum of 74% of the total volume, so the tendency for phase inversion to occur increases. Addition of substances which alter the solubility of an emulsifying agent may also cause phase inversion. The process is irreversible.

Creaming

The term 'creaming' is used to describe the aggregation of globules of the disperse phase at the top or bottom of the emulsion, similar to cream on milk. The process is reversible and gentle shaking redistributes the droplets throughout the continuous phase. Creaming is undesirable because it is inelegant, and inaccurate dosing is possible if shaking is not thorough. Additionally, creaming increases the likelihood of coalescence of globules and therefore the breakdown of the emulsion due to cracking.

Cracking

Cracking is the coalescence of dispersed globules and separation of the disperse phase as a separate layer. It is an irreversible process and redispersion cannot be achieved by shaking.

Causes and prevention of cracking or creaming

- *Globule size.* Stable emulsions require a maximal number of small sized (1–3 µm) globules and as few as possible larger (>15 µm) diameter globules. A homogenizer will efficiently reduce droplet size and may additionally increase the viscosity if more than 30% of disperse phase is present. Homogenizers force the emulsion through a small aperture to reduce the size of the globules
- *Storage temperature.* Extremes of temperature can lead to an emulsion cracking. When water freezes it expands, so undue pressure is exerted on dispersed globules and especially the emulsifying agent film, which may lead to cracking. Conversely, an increased temperature decreases the viscosity of the continuous phase and disrupts the integrity of the interfacial film. An increasing number of collisions between droplets will also occur, leading to increased creaming and cracking
- *Potential for globule coalescence.* Increasing the viscosity of the continuous phase will reduce the potential for globule coalescence as this reduces the movement of globules. Emulsion stabilizers, which increase the viscosity of the continuous phase, may be used in o/w emulsions, e.g. tragacanth, sodium alginate and methylcellulose
- *Changes which affect the interfacial film.* These may be chemical, physical or biological effects: microbiological contamination may destroy the emulsifying agent, especially if a polysaccharide emulsifying agent is being used, addition of a common solvent, addition of an emulsifying agent of opposite charge, for instance cationic to anionic
- Incorporation of excess disperse phase, as discussed above.

Dispensing emulsions

Emulsions can be extemporaneously prepared on a small scale using a mortar and pestle. Electric mixers can also be used, although incorporation of excess air may be a problem. All equipment used must be thoroughly clean and dry. All oil-soluble and water-soluble components of the emulsion are separately dissolved in the appropriate phase. A suitable emulsifying agent must then be used.

Emulsions for oral use

Acacia gum is usually used when making extemporaneous o/w emulsions for oral use, unless otherwise specified. A primary emulsion should be prepared first. This is a thick, stable emulsion prepared using optimal proportions of the ingredients. These vary with the nature of the oil.

Calculating quantities for primary emulsions

Proportions or 'parts' for preparation of primary emulsions are given in Table 7.2. These refer to parts by volume for the different types of oil and water and weight for the acacia gum. If more than one oil is to be incorporated, the quantity of acacia for each is calculated separately and the sum of the quantities used.

Variations to primary emulsion calculations

If the proportion of oil is too small, modifications must be made. Acacia emulsions containing less than 20% oil tend to cream readily. A bland, inert oil, such as sesame, cottonseed or maize oil, should be added to increase the amount of oil.

Methods of preparation of extemporaneous emulsions

There are two possible methods, the dry gum method being the more popular.

Dry gum method of preparation

- Measure the oil accurately in a dry measure. It is important that the measure is dry
- Allow measure to drain into a dry mortar with a large, flat bottom
- Weigh acacia gum

Table 7.2 Quantities for primary emulsions

Type of oil	Examples	Oil	Water	Gum
Fixed	Almond, arachis, cod-liver, castor	4	2	1
Mineral (hydrocarbon)	Liquid paraffin	3	2	1
Volatile	Turpentine, cinnamon, peppermint	2	2	1
Oleo-resin	Male fern extract	1	2	1

- Measure the water for the primary emulsion in a clean measure
- Add acacia to the oil and mix lightly to disperse lumps. Do not over-mix, and keep the suspension in the bottom of the mortar
- Immediately add all of the water (aim to do this within 10–15 s of adding the acacia to the oil) and stir continuously and vigorously until the mixture thickens and the primary emulsion is formed. The mixture thickening, becoming white and producing a 'clicking' sound characterizes this
- Continue mixing for a further 2–3 min to produce the white stable emulsion. The whiter the product, the smaller the globules
- Gradually dilute the primary emulsion with small volumes of the vehicle, ensuring complete mixing between additions
- Gradually add any other ingredients, transfer to a measure and make up to final volume with the vehicle.

Wet gum method of preparation

Water is added to the acacia gum and quickly triturated until the gum has dissolved to make a mucilage. Oil is added to this mucilage in small portions, triturating the mixture thoroughly after each addition until a thick primary emulsion is obtained. The primary emulsion should be stabilized by mixing for several minutes and then completed in the same way as for the dry gum method.

Problems when producing the primary emulsion

The primary emulsion may not form and a thin oily liquid is formed instead. Possible causes are:
- Phase inversion has occurred
- Incorrect quantities of oil or water were used
- There was cross-contamination of water and oil
- A wet mortar was used
- The mortar was too small and curved, or the pestle head was too round, giving insufficient shear
- Excessive mixing of oil and gum before adding water (dry gum method)
- Diluting the primary emulsion too soon
- Too rapid dilution of primary emulsion
- Poor-quality acacia.

Emulsions for external use

Liquid or semi-liquid emulsions may be used as applications, liniments and lotions (see Ch. 8). The extemporaneous preparation of emulsions for external use does not require the preparation of a primary emulsion. Soaps are commonly used as the emulsifying agent and some are prepared 'in situ' by mixing the oily phase containing a fatty acid and the aqueous phase containing the alkali. Alternatively, the emulsifying agent can be dissolved in the oily or aqueous phase and the disperse phase added to the continuous phase, either gradually or in one portion.

Creams are semi-solid emulsions which may be o/w (e.g. aqueous cream) or w/o (e.g. oily cream). (These are considered in more detail in Ch. 8.)

Shelf-life and storage

Emulsions should be stored at room temperature and will either be recently or freshly prepared. Some official preparations will have specific expiry dates. They should not be frozen.

Containers

An amber medicine bottle is used with an airtight child-resistant closure.

Special labelling and advice for emulsions

- 'Shake well before use'
- 'Store in a cool place'. This is to protect the emulsion against extremes of temperature which will adversely affect its stability
- Expiry date
- 'For external use only', for external emulsions.

Worked examples

Example 7.1 **Prepare 200 mL Cod-Liver Oil Emulsion to the following formula:**

Cod-liver oil	60 mL
Chloroform	0.4 mL
Cinnamon water	to 200 mL

Formulation notes. Cod-liver oil is a fixed oil that requires the addition of acacia gum as an emulsifying agent. The proportions are: 4 oil; 2 water; 1 gum. Therefore 60 mL cod-liver oil, 30 mL of cinnamon water and 15 g of acacia gum will be used to prepare the primary emulsion. Cinnamon water acts as a flavouring agent and vehicle. It may need to be prepared from concentrated cinnamon water, at a dilution of 1 part to 39 parts of water. Since 60 mL of the emulsion is the cod-liver oil, it is not necessary to prepare 200 mL of cinnamon water, so 160 mL is adequate. Therefore 4 mL of concentrated cinnamon water will be diluted to 160 mL with water.

Chloroform is dense and only slowly soluble and acts as a preservative.

Method of preparation. Use the dry gum method. Weigh 15 g of acacia, measure 60 mL of cod-liver oil and 30 mL of cinnamon water, which will be used to create the primary emulsion. Place the cod-liver oil in a dry, flat-bottomed mortar. Add the acacia and mix very lightly and briefly. Immediately add the cinnamon water, mixing vigorously until a clicking sound is heard and a white primary emulsion is formed. Continue mixing for a few minutes to stabilize the primary emulsion. Scrape the mortar and pestle with a spatula to ensure that all the oil is incorporated. Add the chloroform by pipette and mix thoroughly. Gradually add most of the remainder of the cinnamon water to the emulsion in the mortar, stirring well between additions. Transfer the emulsion to a 200-mL measure, rinsing the mortar with cinnamon water, adding these washings to the measure. Make up to volume with cinnamon water and pack in an amber medicine bottle with a child-resistant closure.

Storage. Store in a cool, dry place.

Example 7.2 **Prepare 100 mL Liquid Paraffin Oral Emulsion BP 1968.**

Liquid paraffin	50 mL
Vanillin	50 mg
Chloroform	0.25 mL
Benzoic acid solution	2 mL
Methylcellulose 20	2 g
Saccharin sodium	5 mg
Water	to 100 mL

Formulation notes. Methylcellulose 20 at a concentration of 2% acts as an emulsifying agent for the mineral oil, liquid paraffin. A primary emulsion is not required. Benzoic acid and chloroform act as preservatives and vanillin and saccharin sodium act as flavouring and sweetening agent respectively. The amount of saccharin sodium is not weighable on a dispensing balance and will be obtained by trituration using water as the diluent (since this is the vehicle for the emulsion).

Trituration for saccharin sodium:

Saccharin sodium	100 mg
Water	to 100 mL
5 mL of water will contain	5 mg of saccharin sodium

Method of preparation. First, prepare a mucilage by mixing the methylcellulose 20 with about six times its weight of boiling water and allow to stand for 30 minutes to hydrate. Add an equal weight (about 15 g) of ice and stir mechanically until the mucilage is homogeneous. Dissolve the vanillin in the benzoic acid solution and chloroform. Add this mixture to the mucilage and stir for 5 min. Make up the saccharin sodium trituration and stir in the appropriate volume of solution to the mucilage. Make the volume of the mucilage up to 50 mL, taking care to ensure that there is no entrapped air in the mucilage. Make the emulsion by mixing together 50 mL of liquid paraffin and 50 mL of prepared mucilage with constant stirring. The emulsion is more stable if passed through a hand homogenizer. Pack in an amber medicine bottle with a child-resistant closure. Shake well to ensure that the emulsion is thoroughly mixed. Polish and label the bottle and give a 5-mL medicine spoon with the medicine.

Storage. Store in a cool, dry place.

Example 7.3 **Prepare 100 mL Oily Calamine Lotion BP 1980.**

Calamine	5 g
Wool fat	1 g
Oleic acid	0.5 mL
Arachis oil	50 mL
Calcium hydroxide solution	to 100 mL

Formulation notes. The emulsifying agent for the arachis oil is the soap calcium oleate produced from the calcium hydroxide and oleic acid when they are shaken together. Wool fat is included as an emulsion stabilizer. This is a w/o emulsion.

Method of preparation. The wool fat, oleic acid and arachis oil should be warmed gently together in an evaporating basin (using a water bath or heating block) until melted. Mix them thoroughly. The calamine should be sieved and weighed and placed on a warm ointment tile. Add a little of the oily mixture and rub in with a large spatula until smooth. Gradually add more of the oily mixture until it is fluid. Transfer back to the evaporating basin and stir to evenly distribute the calamine powder. Pour into a previously tared, amber ribbed bottle and add the calcium hydroxide solution to the bottle in small amounts, shaking well between additions. Make up to volume and seal with a child-resistant closure. Polish and label the bottle.

Storage. Store in a cool, dry place.

Key points

- Emulsions may be oil-in-water (o/w) or water-in-oil (w/o)
- Emulsions may be used orally, externally or by intramuscular and intravenous injection
- Oral emulsions are always o/w
- The type of emulsion may be determined by miscibility, conductivity, staining and dye tests
- Emulsifying agents are required to reduce the interfacial tension and act as a barrier between the oil and water phases
- Naturally occurring emulsifying agents include polysaccharides (acacia), semi-synthetic polysaccharides (methylcellulose) and sterols (wool fat)
- Synthetic surfactants can be used and are selected using the HLB number
- Care is required to avoid anion–cation incompatibilities
- Some finely divided solids will stabilize emulsions
- Emulsions require antimicrobial preservation
- Phase inversion, creaming and cracking are instabilities of emulsions which must be avoided
- A primary emulsion is prepared when making an emulsion using acacia as the emulsifying agent using either the 'dry gum' or 'wet gum' method
- The ratio of oil:water:acacia used for the primary emulsion will vary with the type of oil in the formulation
- Liquid emulsions should have 'Shake well before use' and 'Store in a cool place' labels and should not be frozen

Chapter 8

External preparations

Arthur J. Winfield

STUDY POINTS

- Skin structure and sites of action of drugs
- The types and functions of solid, liquid and semi-solid skin preparations
- The ingredients used in skin preparations
- Dispensing preparations for use on the skin
- Transdermal drug delivery for systemic activity

Introduction

Skin is the largest organ in the body and has three distinct regions. The hypodermis is the innermost and is often called *subcutaneous fat*. The dermis is the bulk of the thickness of the skin and contains blood vessels, nerve fibres, sweat glands and hair follicles. The outermost region is the epidermis, which is made up of several layers. One of these layers is the stratum basale, in which cells divide and as they move towards the surface, they change appearance and function. The outermost layer, the stratum corneum, acts as the skin barrier. It is made up of about 20 layers of dead keratinized cells. The hair follicles and sweat ducts pass through the stratum corneum to reach the surface. A simplified diagram showing the main skin structures is given in Fig. 8.1.

There are many diseases which may affect different regions of the skin. Any drug used will need to reach the site of the disease in order to act. Unless it is for a surface effect only, the drug must either pass through the stratum corneum or go through hair follicles or sweat ducts. Examples of drugs applied to the skin and their sites of action are shown in Fig. 8.1. Once in the skin, a lipid-soluble drug will tend to accumulate in lipid regions, while more water-soluble drugs will tend to enter the blood capillaries and be

removed from the skin. There are also many metabolic enzymes in the skin which can deactivate drugs.

Effective formulation makes it possible to achieve adequate and reproducible percutaneous absorption, which is close to zero order kinetics. As a consequence, absorption through the skin from toxic materials is possible and so gloves should always be worn when preparing external preparations.

There are an increasing number of drugs that are effective against skin diseases, but drugs are not the only way of treating skin conditions. Creating physiological changes in the skin can also be beneficial. The main change is to control the moisture content of the skin. Normal skin has 10–25% moisture in the stratum corneum. This level may be reduced in, for example, eczema, or increased, as in skin maceration between the toes. By using an occlusive product (that is, an oily product), water leaving the body through the skin will be trapped and the moisture content will increase. These products are called *emollients*. An excess of moisture may be removed using an astringent, a hygroscopic material or, to a lesser extent, a dusting powder. Where an oily vehicle is needed, but moisture must not increase, adding solid particles to the vehicle will allow water to escape. Lubrication of sensitive skin is achieved by using finely divided solids, applied either as a powder or, more efficiently, as a suspension. Cooling the skin relieves inflammation and eases discomfort. It is achieved by evaporating a solvent, usually water or a water and alcohol mixture. Volatile solvents sprayed on the skin give intense cooling.

Types of skin preparation

There are a large number of different types of external medicine, ranging from dry powders through semi-solids

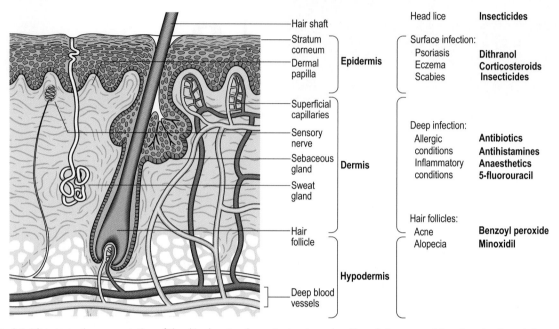

Fig. 8.1 Diagrammatic representation of the skin showing the main structures, location of diseases and the sites of action of drugs.

to liquids. The names are often traditional making classification difficult. Fig. 8.2 illustrates the formulation of the main types of preparation used on the skin.

Solids

Dusting powders are applied to the skin for a surface effect such as drying or lubricating, or an antibacterial action. They are made of a fine-particle-size powder, which may be a drug alone or together with excipients.

Liquids

Soaks have an active ingredient dissolved in an aqueous solvent and are often used as astringents, for cooling or to leave a film of solid on the skin. Oily vehicles can be used in bath additives to leave an emollient film on the skin surface.

Lotions are aqueous solutions, suspensions (see Example 8.1) or emulsions that cool inflamed skin and deposit a protective layer of solid.

Liniments are alcoholic or oily solutions or emulsions (see Example 8.2) designed to be rubbed into the skin. The medicament is usually a rubefacient.

Applications are solutions or emulsions that frequently contain parasiticides (see Example 8.3).

Paints and *tinctures* are concentrated aqueous or alcoholic antimicrobial solutions.

Collodions are organic solvents containing a polymer and drug.

There are also many other liquid products including shampoos and foot washes.

Semi-solids

Ointments are usually oily vehicles that may contain a surfactant to allow them to be washed off easily (barrier creams). They are used as emollients, or for drug delivery either to the surface or for deeper penetration.

Creams are traditionally oil-in-water (o/w) emulsions while *oily creams* are water-in-oil (w/o) emulsions. However, there are also 'creams' that are not emulsions. Emulsified creams usually give cooling, are less greasy than ointments and can be used for drug delivery onto or into the skin. They require antimicrobial preservatives.

Pastes are vehicles (aqueous or oily) with a high concentration of added solid. This makes them thick so they do not spread and so localize drug delivery (e.g. Dithranol in Lassar's paste, see Example 8.9). They can also be used for sun blocks.

Gels are usually aqueous gels used for lubrication or applying a drug to the skin. Oily gels are also available where occlusion is required.

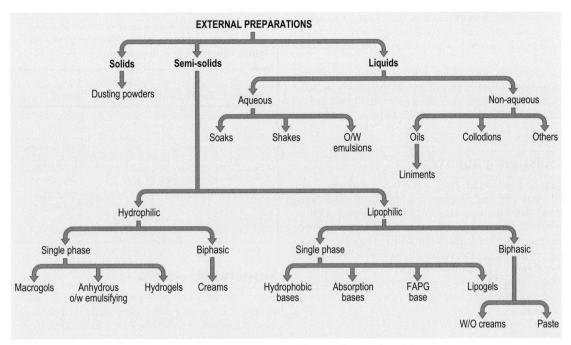

Fig. 8.2 Schematic representation of types of external medicines.

Ingredients used in skin preparations

Water-miscible vehicles

These include water, alcohol and the macrogols. Alcohol, usually industrial denatured alcohol, is often added to water to increase the rate of evaporation and produce a more intense cooling effect. The macrogols (polyethylene glycols) are available with a range of molecular weights. As chain length increases, so the properties change from liquid, through semi-solid to waxy solid. They have good solvent properties for a wide range of drugs and can be blended to produce intermediate consistencies. They tend to dry the skin, inactivate some antimicrobials, interact with some plastics and can give poor release of drugs.

Oily vehicles

Oils used in external preparations come from one of three sources.

Mineral oils (paraffins) are the most widely used. They are complex mixtures of mainly saturated hydrocarbons, which are available in different fractions. Different names are used in different pharmacopoeias (Table 8.1).

Light liquid paraffin is not normally used in external medicines. Soft paraffin is the main ingredient in many

Table 8.1 Paraffins used in external preparations: the names used are different in the UK, USA and European pharmacopoeias

UK	USA	European
Light liquid paraffin	Light mineral oil	Paraffinium perliquidum
Liquid paraffin	Mineral oil	Paraffinium liquidum
Soft paraffin	Petrolatum	Paraffinium molle
Hard paraffin	Paraffin	Paraffinium durum

products, with liquid or hard paraffin being used to thin or thicken them respectively. There are two forms of soft paraffin: yellow and white. The latter has been bleached, residues of which may remain. As a general rule, white is used with white or pale coloured ingredients, while yellow is used for darker ingredients. The paraffins are occlusive and chemically inert, but do not give good skin penetration. It should be noted that these products are flammable and patients should be counselled about the potential risk.

Vegetable oils come from plant sources such as castor, olive, peanut and coconut. The latter two would be rarely used because of severe reactions in patients with nut allergies.

Synthetic oils, such as the silicone oils (Dimethicone BP), are used as water repellents and occlusives because they are very hydrophobic. The semi-synthetic isopropyl-myristate is similar to vegetable oil in its properties and use.

Emulsifying agents

Liquid and semi-solid emulsions, both o/w and w/o, are used externally and require the addition of emulsifying agents. The latter may also be added to an oil without water as in Emulsifying Ointment BP. The presence of a surfactant usually increases the skin penetration of any drug. A wide range of materials can be used as surfactants, either alone or in combinations. Selection is made in view of the type of emulsion required (o/w or w/o) and the charge on the other ingredients (anionic, cationic or non-ionic).

Emulsifiers – w/o

Hypoallergenic commercial wool fat is a complex mixture of fatty acid esters of cholesterol and other sterols and alcohols. Wool alcohol, a solid, is richer in cholesterol and lanosterol and has fewer impurities. Both it and wool fat increase the 'water-holding' capacity of greasy bases. Hydrous wool fat is 7 parts wool fat and 3 parts water and is a softer material. Beeswax is a traditional w/o emulsifier which is occasionally used.

Emulsifiers – o/w

Emulsifying waxes each contain two ingredients: cetostearyl alcohol and a surface-active agent, as shown in Table 8.2. All three bases are waxy solids that mix with oily materials. Addition of water produces an o/w emulsion – a cream. Both the non-aqueous blends and the creams are easily washed off the skin. Varying the amount of bodying agent, usually cetostearyl alcohol, can control consistency. The ratio of oil to water will also alter the consistency of a cream.

Other emulsifiers

Calcium soaps and soft soap have traditionally been used to make o/w emulsions.

Synthetic surface-active agents are used particularly in commercial products. Low hydrophilic–lipophilic balance (HLB) materials will produce w/o emulsions, while higher HLB surfactants give o/w emulsions.

Table 8.2 The ingredients used in the emulsifying waxes described in the *British Pharmacopoeia* (BP) and *British Pharmaceutical Codex* (BPC)

Charge	Surfactant	CSA:SAA ratio	Name
Anionic	Sodium lauryl sulphate	9:1	Emulsifying Wax BP
Cationic	Cetrimide	9:1	Cetrimide Emulsifying Wax BPC
Non-ionic	Cetomacrogol 1000	8:2	Cetomacrogol Emulsifying Wax BPC

CSA, Cetostearyl alcohol; *SAA*, surface active agent.

Suspending agents

These materials can be used for suspending solids in lotions, or to produce gels, depending on the concentration used. Examples are the clays, of which there are many forms, including bentonite, attapulgite, montmorillonite and Veegum (aluminium magnesium silicate). They leave a lubricant layer of powder on the skin. They are unsuitable for use below pH 3.5 and their consistency may be affected by alcohol and electrolytes (see Example 8.5).

Gelling agents can be used to produce a wide range of consistency from slightly thickened (as in artificial tears), through lubricants and semi-solids for the delivery of drugs to very thick bases used to immobilize the skin. For aqueous gels the materials used include tragacanth, alginates, pectin, gelatin, methylcelluloses, carbomer, polyvinyl alcohol and clays. Oils may be thickened using cetostearyl alcohol, hard paraffin, beeswax, wool alcohols and polyvalent soaps such as magnesium stearate. The latter, when heated with an oil, produces a clear 'lipogel'.

Other ingredients

Wetting agents are required for hydrophobic solids. Tincture of quillaia is the traditional material (see Example 8.1), but alcohol alone may be effective. Synthetic materials, such as Manoxol OT, can also be used.

Humectants are materials added to reduce the rate of water loss from creams and gels. They are all hygroscopic materials and include glycerol, propylene glycol, PEG 300 and sorbitol syrup, typically used at concentrations of 5–15%.

Solids may be added to semi-solid occlusive bases. They provide channels for the migration of water from the skin surface and so reduce the occlusiveness. Solids used include zinc oxide, talc, starch and Aerosil. Some, such as talc, must be sterilized to kill bacterial spores.

Whenever there is a danger of microbial growth, antimicrobial preservation is required.

Preparation of external preparations

A wide range of dispensing techniques are used in compounding external medicines, some of which have been reviewed in other chapters (see Chs 2, 5, 6, 7 and 10). In the section that follows, only those types of product which require different dispensing techniques are described in detail.

Dusting powders

A simple mixing in a mortar and pestle using 'doubling-up' is used (see Ch. 10). Sieving may be necessary to disperse aggregates of cohesive powders. A 180µm sieve should be used. Powders such as starch, which contains a lot of moisture, may need drying to ensure optimum flow properties. With coloured materials, considerable working with the pestle is required before proceeding to 'doubling-up', otherwise a speckled product may result. A liquid may be added by pipette to a small quantity of the powder and be worked in before further mixing. A worked example of a dusting powder is given in Example 10.3.

Liquid preparations

These include solutions, suspensions and emulsion. Most liquid preparations are used unsterilized, but if they are intended for application to broken skin, eyes or body cavities, they should be sterilized. They should be labelled 'For external use only', and carry a 'Shake the bottle' label if they are emulsions or suspensions. Worked examples are given, of a lotion in Example 6.3 and of an oily lotion in Example 7.3.

Example 8.1 **Prepare 100 mL Compound Sulphur Lotion BPC.**

	Master formula	For 100 mL
Precipitated sulphur	40 g	4 g
Quillaia tincture	5 mL	0.5 mL
Glycerol	20 mL	2 mL
Industrial denatured alcohol	60 mL	6 mL
Calcium hydroxide solution	to 1000 mL	to 100 mL

Formulation notes. This an example of a 'shake' lotion, an aqueous suspension prepared without a suspending agent, but including a wetting agent for the hydrophobic sulphur.

Method of preparation. Sieve the precipitated sulphur. Weigh out 4 g and place in a glass mortar. Using a 1-mL pipette, add 0.5 mL quillaia tincture and work well into the sulphur using a pestle. Add 6 mL of industrial methylated spirits followed by 2 mL glycerol, working in after each addition (thus achieving maximum wetting before water is added). Add 20–30 mL calcium hydroxide solution to produce a pourable suspension. Transfer to a tared bottle. Rinse the mortar with calcium hydroxide solution, adding it to the bottle, before making up to volume.

Shelf-life and storage. There are no special requirements for storage. An expiry date of 4 weeks is suitable.

Example 8.2 **Prepare 100 mL Methyl Salicylate Liniment BP.**

	Master formula	For 100 mL
Methyl salicylate	250 mL	25 mL
Arachis oil	to 1000 mL	to 100 mL

Formulation notes. The methyl salicylate requires to penetrate the skin. The vegetable oil, arachis oil, is used as the solvent to assist in the penetration of the skin by methyl salicylate. Other similar fixed oils can be used.

Method of preparation. Measure 25 mL of methyl salicylate in a 100-mL measure and add arachis oil to make up to volume. Transfer to a dry 100-mL amber ribbed bottle.

Shelf-life and storage. This liniment should be kept in a well-closed container in a cool place. An expiry date of 4 weeks is appropriate.

Example 8.3 **Prepare 100 mL of Benzyl Benzoate Application BP.**

	Master formula	For 100 mL
Benzyl benzoate	250 g	25 g
Emulsifying wax	20 g	2 g
Purified water, freshly boiled and cooled	to 1000 mL	to 100 mL

Formulation notes. Benzyl benzoate is water immiscible and is being emulsified using the anionic Emulsifying Wax BP. The application is an o/w emulsion.

Method of preparation. Weigh the emulsifying wax and place it in an evaporating basin on a water bath or hot plate to melt. Add the benzyl benzoate and mix and warm. Warm about 75 mL of the water to the same temperature. Add about half of this to the evaporating basin and mix very gently. Transfer the mixture, again very gently to avoid frothing, to a tared bottle. Add warmed water to volume. Close the bottle and shake vigorously. Care is required to avoid frothing when water is present, because it will be very difficult to make up to the tare mark when froth has formed. Shake frequently during cooling.

Shelf-life and storage. The application should be kept in a cool place, but not be allowed to freeze. An expiry date of 4 weeks is appropriate.

Semi-solid preparations

Mixing by fusion

The compounding of many semi-solid preparations includes the blending together of oily materials, some of which are solids at room temperature. The process called 'mixing by fusion' achieves this. As the name implies, it involves melting the ingredients together (see Example 8.4). The process is carried out in an evaporating basin on a water bath or hot plate. It should be noted that a high temperature is not required so 60–70 °C is usually adequate. Waxy solids should be grated before weighing and should be added first, so that melting can start while other ingredients are being measured. When all the ingredients are melted, remove the basin from the water bath and gently stir until cold. Mixing, which should be gentle to avoid air bubbles, is necessary to avoid lumps forming. This could happen because the higher melting point ingredients in the eutectic system may precipitate out. Any medicament may be added at different stages of preparation depending on its properties. If soluble and stable, it can be added when the base is molten. If it is less stable, or insoluble but easy to disperse, it can be added during cooling. However, if it is unstable or if dispersion is difficult, it should be added when cold using mixing by trituration.

When evaporating basins are being used, recovery of all the product is not possible. Thus in order to be able to pack the prescribed amount, it is necessary to make an excess of about 10%.

Formulation notes. This is a simple blend of solid and semi-solid oily ingredients made by fusion. Yellow or white soft paraffin is chosen according to the colour of the finished product. In this case, since there is nothing else to be added, white soft paraffin should be used; 60 g is made to allow 50 g to be dispensed.

Method of preparation. Grate the hard paraffin and cetostearyl alcohol. Weigh 3 g of each and place in an evaporating basin on a water bath or hot plate. Weigh the wool fat, using a piece of paper to allow full recovery of the material, and add it to the evaporating basin, followed by the soft paraffin (also weighed on paper). Stir gently until fully melted. Remove from the heat and continue to stir gently until cold. Weigh 50 g of base into a tared ointment jar. If an ointment jar is used, a greaseproof paper disc should be placed on the surface of the ointment to protect the liner of the lid from the greasiness.

Shelf-life and storage. Store in a cool place. An expiry date of 4 weeks is appropriate.

Mixing by trituration

Insoluble solids or liquids are incorporated into bases using the technique called 'mixing by trituration'. Any powders should be passed through a 180-µm sieve before weighing to avoid grittiness in the finished product. Mixing by trituration is carried out on an ointment slab or tile, which may be made of glass or glazed porcelain. A flexible spatula is used to work the materials together. Powders are placed on the tile and incorporated into the base using 'doubling-up' as it is worked in. However, it is usually necessary to have two to three times the volume of base to powder, otherwise it will 'crumble'. Liquids, if present, are usually present in small amounts. To incorporate a liquid, a portion of the base is placed on the slab and a recess made to hold the liquid which is then worked in gently. Larger quantities of liquid should be added a little at a time using the same method. In theory, it is possible to recover all material from the slab, but it is normal to allow up to 10% excess for losses. These processes can be carried out in a mortar with a flat base using a pestle with a flat head. However, because recovery of the product is difficult, this is usually reserved for larger-scale batches.

Example 8.4 **Prepare 50 g of Simple Ointment BP.**

	Master formula	For 60 g
Wool fat	50 g	3 g
Hard paraffin	50 g	3 g
Cetostearyl alcohol	50 g	3 g
Yellow or white soft paraffin	850 g	51 g

Example 8.5 **Prepare 50 g of Sulphur Ointment BP.**

	Master formula	For 50 g	For 55 g
Precipitated sulphur, finely sifted	100 g	5 g	5.5 g
Simple ointment	900 g	45 g	49.5 g

Formulation notes. The BP directs that the simple ointment be prepared with white soft paraffin. If simple ointment is available, the trituration can be carried out on a slab and all the product recovered. However, if simple ointment is also being made, 50 g should be adequate to ensure that 45 g is available. Precipitated sulphur, while of smaller particle size than sublimed sulphur, can give a gritty feel unless it is passed through a 180-μm sieve.

Method of preparation. Sieve and then weigh out the precipitated sulphur and place it on the slab. Weigh out the simple ointment (using a piece of paper to prevent it sticking to the balance), and place it on a different part of the slab. Take a portion of the sulphur and a portion of the base of about three times the volume of the sulphur and work them together vigorously until there is no sign of any particles of sulphur. Spreading a thin layer on the slab helps check this. Gradually add the remaining sulphur and base. Collect the ointment together on the slab using the spatula and pack 50 g.

Shelf-life and storage. Store in a cool place. An expiry date of 4 weeks is appropriate.

Example 8.6 **Prepare 30 g of Methyl Salicylate Ointment BP.**

	Master formula	For 35 g
Methyl salicylate	500 g	17.5 g
White beeswax	250 g	8.75 g
Hydrous wool fat	250 g	8.75 g

Formulation notes. Methyl salicylate is a liquid. With the high proportion present, the product would be runny without the addition of the beeswax as a thickening agent. The base ingredients require to be blended by fusion.

Method of preparation. Grate and weigh the beeswax. Melt it with the hydrous wool fat (weighed on a piece of paper) in an evaporating basin on a water bath or hot plate. Remove from the heat and stir until almost cold before adding the methyl salicylate (it is volatile). Continue stirring until cold. Pack 30 g in a glass ointment jar (plastic should be avoided with methyl salicylate).

Shelf-life and storage. Store in a cool place. An expiry date of 4 weeks is appropriate.

Creams

Creams are emulsified preparations containing water. They are susceptible to microorganisms which may cause spoilage of the cream or disease in the patient. While preservatives are included, they are usually inadequate to cope with a heavy microbial contamination and growth so the possibility of microbial contamination during preparation should be minimized. Ideally aseptic techniques should be used, but this is not normally possible in extemporaneous dispensing and so thorough cleanliness is employed. As a minimum, all apparatus and final containers should be thoroughly cleaned and rinsed with freshly boiled and cooled purified water, then dried just prior to use. Swabbing of working surfaces, spatulas and other equipment with ethanol will also reduce the possibility of microbial contamination.

The basic method of making an emulsified cream is to warm both the oily phase and aqueous phase separately to a temperature of about 60°C, mix the phases and stir until cold. It is important that the temperatures of the two phases are within a few degrees of each other and it is advisable to use a thermometer to check this. Rapid cooling will cause the separation of high melting point materials, and excessive aeration as a result of vigorous stirring will produce a granular appearance in the product. Medicaments may, if they are stable, be dissolved in the appropriate phase before emulsification, or can be added by trituration when cold.

Example 8.7 **Prepare 50 g of Aqueous Cream BP.**

	Master formula	For 55 g
Emulsifying ointment	300 g	16.5 g
Phenoxyethanol	10 g	0.55 g
Purified water, freshly boiled and cooled	690 g	37.95 g

Formulation notes. This is an o/w cream made using an anionic emulsifying agent. To reduce the risk of microbial contamination, all equipment should be washed before use. Phenoxyethanol is present as an antimicrobial preservative. It is a liquid, so has to be weighed, or, if its density is obtained, it could be measured by pipette. If the emulsifying ointment has to be made, exactly 16.5 g can be made because the emulsification can be carried out in the same evaporating basin.

Method of preparation. The phenoxyethanol is dissolved in the water warmed to 60°C. Weigh the emulsifying ointment (using a piece of paper to prevent it sticking) and melt it in an evaporating basin on a water bath or hot plate. Ensure that both phases are close to 60°C, then add the aqueous phase to the melted ointment. Remove from the heat and stir continuously until cold, taking care not to incorporate too much air. Weigh 50 g and pack in an ointment jar.

Shelf-life and storage. The preparation should be stored in a cool place, but not allowed to freeze. A shelf-life of 2–3 weeks is appropriate because the preparation has not been made in the cleanest conditions.

Example 8.8 **Prepare 50 g of Hydrous Ointment BP (also known as Oily Cream).**

	Master formula	For 60 g
Wool alcohols ointment	500 g	30 g
Phenoxyethanol	10 g	0.6 g
Dried magnesium sulphate	5 g	0.3 g
Purified water, freshly boiled and cooled	485 g	29.1 g

Formulation notes. This is a w/o cream prepared using wool alcohols as the emulsifying agent. Phenoxyethanol is present as preservative, but all equipment should be washed before use. Phenoxyethanol is a liquid and so must be weighed, or, if its density is obtained, it can be measured by pipette. Quantities for 55 g produce amounts that cannot be weighed on a dispensing balance, so 60 g is made. If the wool alcohols ointment is also to be made, exactly 30 g is adequate, because it does not have to be removed from the evaporating basin.

Method of preparation. All equipment should be thoroughly cleaned before use. Dissolve the magnesium sulphate and phenoxyethanol in the water and warm to 60°C on a water bath or hot plate. Weigh the wool alcohols ointment, using a piece of paper, and melt it in an evaporating basin at 60°C. Check that the two temperatures are the same. Add the water, little by little, to the ointment, stirring constantly until a smooth creamy mixture is produced, while maintaining the temperature at 60°C. When all the water is added, remove from the heat and stir gently until the cream is at room temperature. Pack 50 g in an ointment jar.

Shelf-life and storage. Store in a cool place but do not allow to freeze. If liquid separates on storage, stirring may reincorporate it. An expiry date of 4 weeks is appropriate.

Dilution of creams

It is sometimes necessary to prepare a dilution of a commercially produced cream, although the practice is undesirable. Choice of diluent is crucial, since the diluent may impair the preservative system in the cream, may affect the bioavailability of the medicament or may be incompatible with other ingredients. The process of dilution also increases the risk of microbial contamination. Thus dilutions should only be made with the diluent(s) specified in the manufacturer's data sheet and heat must be avoided. All diluted creams should be freshly prepared and be given a 2-week shelf-life.

Pastes

Pastes are dispersions of high concentrations of solid in either an aqueous or oily vehicle. They can be used to treat infections by making use of their high osmotic pressure, or as very thick materials to prevent irritant drugs spreading over the skin surface. Incorporation of the solid is by mixing on an ointment slab.

Example 8.9 **Prepare 100 g of Dithranol Paste BP.**

	Master formula	For 100 g
Dithranol	1 g	0.1 g
Lassar's paste	999 g	99.9 g
Lassar's paste	Master formula	For 110 g
Zinc oxide	240 g	26.4 g
Salicylic acid	20 g	2.2 g
Starch	240 g	26.4 g
White soft paraffin	500 g	55 g

Formulation notes. The Lassar's paste has to be made first before incorporating the dithranol. Dithranol is prone to oxidation, so contact with metal should be avoided. Gloves should be worn during preparation.

Method of preparation. Sieve the zinc oxide and salicylic acid through a 180-μm sieve before weighing. Weigh the soft paraffin (on a piece of paper) and melt in an evaporating basin on a water bath. Take some of the powder and stir into the melted base. Continue until all the powder is added, then stir gently until cold. Weigh out the Lassar's paste (using paper to avoid sticking). Only when the Lassar's paste has been completed, weigh out the dithranol. Care is required because it is very irritant to skin. Place it on a slab and incorporate it in a small portion of the paste using a plastic spatula, ensuring that a smooth, even product is produced. Dilute gradually with the remainder of the paste. Pack in a brown ointment jar, with a circle of greaseproof paper and a tight-fitting closure.

Shelf-life and storage. The product should be kept in a cool place, protected from light. An expiry date of 2 weeks is appropriate because of chemical instability.

Transdermal delivery systems

Transdermal drug delivery systems aim to provide continuous drug release over a period of time which can be from a few hours to 7 days.

The principle of this dosage form is that, by optimization of physicochemical factors, the drug is absorbed through the skin into the systemic circulation. Absorption through the skin is variable so the rate of release of the drug must be controlled to a slower rate than the skin can absorb it. This may be achieved either by using a matrix system or a rate-limiting membrane. These devices are commonly known as 'patches'. Drugs available as transdermal therapeutic systems include glyceryl trinitrate, oestradiol, nicotine, hyoscine, testosterone, fentanyl, rivastigmine. Transdermal therapeutic systems are always produced by pharmaceutical manufacturers because of the technology involved.

Advantages

- Continuous drug delivery, producing steady-state plasma levels
- No drug deactivation in the gastrointestinal tract
- No first pass effect, as the liver is bypassed (although there is metabolism in the skin)
- Cessation of treatment by removing the patch. (This is not immediate because of a reservoir effect which will continue to deliver drug from the skin for several hours.)

Although these are benefits, various problems are associated with this type of dosage form. For these reasons, few drugs so far have been formulated in this way.

Disadvantages

- Only potent drugs, i.e. those with a small therapeutic dose, are suitable to be incorporated into a patch. Skin permeability is inadequate to allow larger doses from an acceptable size of patch
- Because the drug is being absorbed through the skin, lipid-soluble drugs are most likely to be effective
- Drugs with long half-lives are not suitable for this type of formulation
- There have been reports of local skin reactions due to irritancy by drugs. To minimize possible skin reactions, new patches should be placed on fresh skin each time, the same site being not used for at least 7 days
- In some instances, the steady-state blood levels have produced tolerance, e.g. glyceryl trinitrate. This has led to the practice of patients being given a 'nitrate-free' period which prevents tolerance occurring
- Steady-state blood levels of nicotine have caused central nervous system disturbance; in particular, patients have reported suffering nightmares. Normally, nicotine levels in a smoker will fall during the hours of sleep as no cigarette smoking occurs. No such fall will

occur when 24-hour nicotine patches are used. For this reason, manufacturers have developed patches which are applied for 16 hours then removed. A new one is applied 8 hours later.

Method of use

It is important that patients are informed how to use patches correctly. All patients who purchase or are prescribed patches should be given the following information about their use:

- To ensure adequate adhesion, the patch must be applied to a clean, dry area of skin. Ideally the patch will not be applied to a very hairy area of skin, due to pain on removal of the patch
- The old patch must always be removed before applying a new one
- When a patch is replaced with a new one it must be applied to a different area of skin. The area of skin from which a patch has just been removed will be soft and possibly moist. This alters the permeability of the skin. In order to maintain the same level of drug absorption, a different, intact area of skin must be used
- The patch must be disposed of carefully. It should be folded together to prevent it being stuck on to another person's skin. Particular care should be taken to keep patches away from children.

Key points

- Drugs applied to the skin are usually for a local effect, although systemic action is possible
- Skin preparations may be solids, liquids or semi-solids
- For liquids and semi-solids, the vehicles may be water based, water miscible, oily or emulsified
- A wide range of emulsifying agents may be used to produce either o/w or w/o emulsions
- Suspending agents used on the skin are usually clays
- Other ingredients include wetting agents, humectants and finely divided solids
- All skin preparations should carry the label 'For external use only'
- Dusting powders are simple mixtures made by 'doubling-up'
- Lotions are aqueous solutions, suspensions or emulsions
- Liniments are oily solutions or emulsions
- Mixing by fusion is the process of melting together the ingredients of ointment bases followed by stirring until cold

- Mixing by trituration is the incorporation of solids or liquids into semi-solid vehicles on an ointment slab
- Cleanliness is essential when making creams to avoid excessive microbial contamination

- Transdermal delivery systems (skin patches) are used to give prolonged constant plasma concentrations for a number of drugs
- Patients must be carefully counselled on the use of skin patches

Chapter | 9 |

Suppositories and pessaries

Arthur J. Winfield

STUDY POINTS

- Ideal suppository bases
- Types of base
- Suppository moulds and mould calibration
- Displacement values
- Methods of preparation of suppositories and pessaries
- Containers, labelling and patient advice for suppositories and pessaries

Introduction

Drug administration by the rectum can be used for local or systemic action. Dosage forms used include suppositories, rectal tablets, capsules, ointments and enemas. Vaginal administration can be for both local and systemic action, using pessaries and vaginal formulations of tablets, capsules, solutions, sprays, creams, ointments and foams. This chapter gives details of how suppositories and pessaries are prepared extemporaneously, the substances and equipment used in their preparation, the calculations involved and patient advice.

Suppositories and pessaries are drug delivery systems where the drug is incorporated into an inert vehicle; the base. Suppositories are formed by melting the base, incorporating the drug and then allowing them to set in a suitable metal or plastic mould.

Suppository bases

A number of criteria can be identified as desirable in an ideal base, including:

- Melt at, or just below, body temperature or dissolve in body fluids
- Solidify quickly after melting
- Easily moulded and removed from the mould
- Chemically stable even when molten
- Release the active ingredient readily
- Easy to handle
- Bland, i.e. non-toxic and non-irritant.

No base meets all these requirements, so a compromise is required. There are two groups of materials, the fatty bases and the water-soluble or water-miscible bases.

The fatty bases

Theobroma oil

Theobroma oil, a naturally occurring oil, has a melting point range of 30–36°C and so readily melts in the body. It liquefies easily on heating but sets rapidly when cooled. It is also bland and therefore no irritation occurs. The main technical difficulty is the ease with which lower melting point polymorphic forms of theobroma oil are formed. The stable β-form has a melting point of 34.5°C and forms after melting at 36°C and slowly cooling. If it is overheated, the unstable α-form (melting point 23°C) and γ-form (melting point 19°C) are produced. These forms will eventually return to the stable form but this may take several days. The melting point is a problem in hot climates and can be reduced further by the addition of a soluble drug. The latter effect can be counteracted by adding beeswax (up to 10%), but care must be taken not to raise the melting point too high, as the suppository would not melt in the rectum. In addition, theobroma oil is prone to oxidation. Theobroma oil shrinks only slightly on cooling and therefore tends to stick to the suppository mould; thus requiring a mould lubricant.

Synthetic fats

These are hydrogenated vegetable oils. Synthetic fatty bases have many of the advantages but there are a few potential problems:

- The viscosity of the melted fats is lower than that of theobroma oil. As a result, there is a greater risk of drug particles sedimenting during preparation leading to a lack of uniform drug distribution. This problem is partly compensated for in that these bases set very quickly
- These bases become brittle if cooled too rapidly, so should not be refrigerated during preparation
- These bases are produced in series of grades, each with different hardness and melting point ranges. These can be used to compensate for melting point reduction by soluble drugs. However, release and absorption of the drug in the body may vary depending on the base being used.

Further information on these bases can be found in the *Pharmaceutical Codex* (1994).

Water-soluble and water-miscible bases

Glycerol-gelatin bases

These bases are a mixture of glycerol and water stiffened with gelatin. The commonest is Glycerol Suppositories Base BP, which has 14% weight in weight (w/w) gelatin, and 70% w/w glycerol. In hot climates, the gelatin content can be increased to 18% w/w. Pharmaceutical grade gelatin is a pathogen-free, purified protein produced by the hydrolysis of the collagenous tissue, such as skins and bones, of animals. Some people may have ethical problems with the use of such a product.

Two types of gelatin are used for pharmaceutical purposes: Type A, which is prepared by acid hydrolysis and is cationic, and Type B, which is prepared by alkaline hydrolysis and is anionic. Type A is compatible with substances such as boric acid and lactic acid, while Type B is compatible with substances like ichthammol and zinc oxide. The 'jelly strength' or 'bloom strength' of gelatin is important, particularly when it is used in the preparation of suppositories or pessaries.

Glycerol-gelatin bases have a physiological effect which can cause rectal irritation because of the small amount of liquid present. As they dissolve in the mucous secretions of the rectum, osmosis occurs producing a laxative effect. The solution time depends on the content, quality of the gelatin and the age of the suppository. Because of the water content, microbial contamination is more likely than with the fatty bases. Preservatives may be added to the product, but can lead to problems of incompatibility. In addition, glycerol-gelatin bases are hygroscopic and therefore require careful storage.

Macrogols

These polyethylene glycols can be blended together to produce suppository bases with varying melting points, dissolution rates and physical characteristics. Drug release depends on the base dissolving rather than melting (the melting point is often around 50 °C). Higher proportions of high molecular weight polymers produce preparations which release the drug slowly and are also brittle. Less brittle products which release the drug more readily can be prepared by mixing high polymers with medium and low polymers. Details of combinations which are used are found in the *Pharmaceutical Codex* (1994). Macrogols have several properties which make them useful as suppository bases including the absence of a physiological effect, are not prone to microbial contamination and have a high water-absorbing capacity. As they dissolve, a viscous solution is produced which means there is less likelihood of leakage from the body.

The macrogol bases have a number of disadvantages. They are hygroscopic, which means they must be carefully stored, and this could lead to irritation of the rectal mucosa. This latter disadvantage can be alleviated by dipping the suppository in water prior to insertion. They become brittle if cooled too quickly and also may become brittle on storage. Incompatibility with several drugs and packaging materials, e.g. benzocaine and plastic, may limit their use. In addition, crystal growth occurs, with some drugs causing irritation to the rectal mucosa and may prolong dissolution times.

Preparation of suppositories

Suppositories are made using a metal or plastic suppository mould. Traditional metal moulds (Fig. 9.1) are in two halves which are clamped together with a screw. The internal surface is normally plated to ensure that the suppositories have a smooth surface.

Before use, the mould should be completely cleaned by washing carefully in warm, soapy water and thoroughly dried, taking care not to scratch the internal surface. The exact shape can vary slightly from one mould to another.

Preparation of suppositories containing an active ingredient which is insoluble in the base

The bases most commonly used for extemporaneous preparation of suppositories and pessaries are the synthetic fats and glycerol-gelatin base.

1. When calculating the quantity of ingredients, it is necessary to prepare excess due to unavoidable wastage.

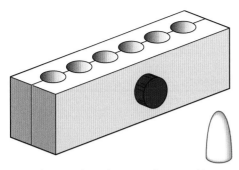

Fig. 9.1 Dispensing suppository mould.

Table 9.1 Lubricants for use with suppository bases

Base	Lubricant
Theobroma oil	Soap spirit
Glycerol-gelatin base	Almond oil, liquid paraffin
Synthetic fats	No lubricant required
Macrogols	No lubricant required

Usually, an excess of two should be calculated for, e.g. to prepare 12 suppositories, calculate for 14.

2. The mould should be carefully washed and dried.
3. Ensure that the two halves fit together correctly. This is necessary to ensure that there is no leakage of material. They usually have code letters and/or numbers which should match.
4. For some bases, the mould will need to be lubricated. The lubricants are given in Table 9.1.
5. If a lubricant is necessary, apply it carefully to the two halves of the mould using gauze or other non-fibrous material. Do not use cotton wool as fibres may be left on the mould surface and become incorporated into the suppositories.
6. Invert the mould to allow any excess lubricant to drain off.
7. Accurately weigh the required amount of base. If large lumps are present, the material should be grated.
8. Place in a porcelain basin and warm gently using a water bath or hot plate. Allow approximately two-thirds of the base to melt and remove from the heat. The residual heat will be sufficient to melt the rest of the base.
9. Reduce the particle size of the active ingredient, if necessary. Either grinding in a mortar and pestle or sieving (see Ch. 2).
10. Weigh the correct amount of medicament and place on a glass tile (ointment slab).
11. Add about half of the molten base to the powdered drug and rub together with a spatula.
12. Scrape the dispersion off the tile using the spatula and place it back in the basin.
13. If necessary, put the basin back over the water bath to remelt the ingredients.
14. Remove from the heat and stir constantly until almost on the point of setting. If the mixture is not stirred at this stage the active ingredient will sediment and uniform distribution of the drug will not be achieved.
15. Quickly pour into the mould, slightly overfilling each cavity to allow for contraction on cooling. Do not start pouring the suppositories while the mixture is still very molten. If this is done, a suspended drug will sediment to the bottom of the mould and the base shrinks excessively so that the tops become concave.
16. Leave the mould and its contents to cool for about 5 min and then, using a spatula, trim the tops of the suppositories. Do not leave the suppositories too long before trimming, as they will be too hard and trimming becomes very difficult.
17. Allow cooling for another 10–15 min until the suppositories are completely firm and set. Do not try to speed up the cooling process by putting the mould in a refrigerator. Synthetic fats in particular are inclined to become brittle and break if cooled too quickly.
18. Unscrew the mould and remove the suppositories.
19. Each perfect suppository should then be wrapped in greaseproof paper and packed in an appropriate container and labelled.

When preparing suppositories where the active ingredient is either a semi-solid, is soluble in the base or is a liquid which is miscible with the base, the melting point of the base will be lowered. In these situations, a base with a higher than normal melting point should be used if available. The base is melted as normal and the active ingredient is added directly to the base and incorporated by stirring.

Moulds are made in four sizes: 1 g, 2 g, 4 g and 8 g. Unless otherwise stated, the 1-g size is used for suppositories. The same moulds are used to prepare pessaries, when the two larger sizes are generally used. A suppository mould is filled by volume, but the suppository is formulated by weight. The capacity of a suppository mould is nominal and each mould will have minor variations. Therefore the weight of material contained in different moulds may be different and will also depend on the base being used. It is therefore essential that each mould be calibrated for each different base.

Mould calibration

The capacity of the mould is confirmed by filling the mould with the chosen base. The total weight of the perfect suppositories is taken and a mean weight calculated. This value is the calibration value of the mould for that particular base (see Example 9.1).

Example 9.1

A 1-g suppository mould is to be used to prepare a batch of suppositories. The base to be used is a synthetic fat. Some base is melted in an evaporating basin over a water bath or hot plate. When about two-thirds of the base has melted, the basin is removed from the heat. The contents of the basin are stirred and the remaining base melts with the residual heat. Continue stirring the base until it is almost on the point of setting (it starts to thicken, becomes slightly cloudy and small crystals can be seen on the surface). The base is then poured into the mould cavities, slightly overfilling to allow for shrinkage. They are trimmed after about 5 min and left to set for a further 10–15 min. The mould is then opened and the suppositories removed. Only the perfect products should be weighed. Any which are chipped or damaged should be discarded.

From the above exercise, five perfect suppositories were obtained. The total weight was 5.05 g. The mould calibration figure is therefore 5.05/5 = 1.01 g. This is the value which should be used for that particular combination of mould and base.

Displacement values

The volume of a suppository from a particular mould is uniform but its weight can vary when a drug is present because the density of the drug may be different from that of the base. For example, a drug which has twice the density of the base will occupy half the volume which the same weight of base occupies, and a drug whose density is four times that of the base will occupy a quarter the volume which the same weight of base occupies. Allowance must be made for this by using displacement values (DV).

The DV of a drug is the number of parts by weight of drug which displaces 1 part by weight of the base.

DV for a variety of medicaments are given in Table 9.2. Other reference sources such as the *Pharmaceutical Handbook* (Wade 1985) and the *Pharmaceutical Codex* also give information on DVs. Minor variations may occur in the values quoted so it is always advisable to indicate the source of your information (see Example 9.2).

DVs in the literature normally refer to values for theobroma oil. These values can also be used for other fatty bases. With glycerol-gelatin suppository base, approximately 1.2 g occupies the same volume as 1 g of theobroma oil. Using this information, the relevant DVs can be calculated.

There may be occasions when information on the DV of a drug is not available. In these situations, the DV must be determined (see Example 9.3).

Table 9.2 Displacement values with respect to fatty bases

Medicament	Displacement value
Aspirin	1.1
Bismuth subgallate	2.7
Chloral hydrate	1.4
Cinchocaine hydrochloride	1.0
Codeine phosphate	1.1
Hamamelis dry extract	1.5
Hydrocortisone	1.5
Ichthammol	1.0
Liquids	1.0
Metronidazole	1.7
Morphine hydrochloride	1.6
Paracetamol	1.5
Pethidine hydrochloride	1.6
Phenobarbital	1.1
Zinc oxide	4.7

Example 9.2 **Prepare Six Suppositories Each Containing 250 mg Bismuth Subgallate.**

Not all material can be removed from the evaporating basin, so quantities are calculated for an excess of two suppositories. Therefore calculate for eight suppositories.

DV of bismuth subgallate = 2.7 (*Pharmaceutical Codex*), i.e. 2.7 g of bismuth subgallate displaces 1 g of base.

A 1-g mould will be used with mould calibration = 0.94.

To calculate the amount of base required, a simple equation is used:

$$\text{Amount of base} = (N \times y) - (N \times D)/DV$$

where N is the number of suppositories to be made, y is the mould calibration, D is the dose in one suppository, DV is the displacement value.

Using the terms in the equation for this example:

$N = 8$
$Y = 0.94$
$D = 250 \text{ mg} = 0.25 \text{ g}$
$DV = 2.7$

Using the equation:
Amount of base required
$= 8 \times 0.94 - 8 \times 0.25 / 2.7 = 7.52 - 0.741$
$= 6.779 \text{ g} = 6.78 \text{ g}$

Example 9.3 **To Calculate the DV of a Drug**

A batch of unmedicated suppositories is prepared and the products weighed.

A batch of suppositories containing a known concentration of the required drug is prepared and the products are weighed.

Weight of six unmedicated suppositories = 6 g
Weight of six suppositories containing 40% drug = 8.8 g
Weight of base is then = 60% = 60 / 100 × 8.8 = 5.28 g
Weight of drug in suppositories = 40% = 40 / 100 × 8.8 = 3.52
Weight of base displaced by drug = 6 ×5.28 = 0.72 g.
If 0.72 g of drug is displaced by 3.52 g of base, then 1 g of base will be displaced by 3.52/0.72 g = 4.88 g.
Therefore DV of drug = 4.9 (rounded to one decimal place).

Calculation of quantities when the active ingredient is stated as a percentage

A DV is not required when calculating quantities stated as percentages (see Example 9.4).

When there is more than one active ingredient present the quantity of each medicament is calculated and the amount of base is calculated using the DV for each ingredient (see Example 9.5).

Example 9.4 **Prepare Eight Suppositories Containing 18% Zinc Oxide.**

Calculate for 10 suppositories (two excess).
Mould calibration = 1
Weight of base required to fill mould = 10 × 1 = 10
Zinc oxide is 18% of total = 1.8 g
Weight of base required = 10 − 1.8 = 8.2 g

Example 9.5 **Calculate the Quantities Required to Make 15 Suppositories Each Containing 150 Mg Hamamelis Dry Extract and 560 Mg of Zinc Oxide.**

A 2-g mould, with mould calibration of 2.04, will be used.
Calculate for 17 suppositories (two excess).
DV of hamamelis dry extract = 1.5 (*Pharmaceutical Codex*)
DV of zinc oxide = 4.7 (*Pharmaceutical Codex*)
Weight of hamamelis dry extract = 17 × 0.15 = 2.55 g
Weight of zinc oxide = 17 × 0.56 = 9.52 g
Weight of base = 17 × 2.04 − (2.55 / 1.5+ 9.52 / 4.7) = 34.68 − (1.7 + 2.03) = 30.95 g.

Preparation of suppositories using a glycerol-gelatin base

The formula for Glycerol Suppository Base BP is:

Gelatin	14%
Glycerol	70%
Water	to 100%

1. The gelatin strip is cut into small pieces, approximately 1 cm square, trimming off any hard outer edges.
2. The required amount of gelatin is weighed and placed in a previously weighed porcelain evaporating basin.
3. Sufficient water to just cover the gelatin is added and the contents left for about 5 min.
4. When the gelatin has softened (hydrated), any excess water is drained off. This step is not necessary if powdered gelatin is being used.
5. The exact amount of glycerol is then weighed into the basin.
6. The basin is heated gently on a water bath or hot plate and the mixture gently stirred until the gelatin has dissolved. Do not stir vigorously as this will create air bubbles which are very difficult to remove. At this stage, the base may need to be heat treated as noted below.
7. When the gelatin is dissolved, the basin is removed from the heat and weighed. If the weight is less than the required total (basin plus ingredients), water is added to give the correct weight. If the contents of the basin are too heavy, it must be heated further to evaporate the excess water.
8. When the correct weight is achieved, the active ingredient is added, with careful stirring.
9. The mixture is then poured into the prepared mould and lubricated with an oil such as almond oil or liquid paraffin. The mould must not be overfilled because glycerol-gelatin base cannot be trimmed.
10. The preparation is left to set. After removing from the mould, each suppository should be smeared with liquid paraffin before being wrapped in greaseproof paper.

Note: Pharmaceutical gelatin should not contain any pathogens, but as a precaution, the base may be heat treated. This is done by heating the base for 1 h at 100°C in an electric steamer. This should be done before the base is adjusted to weight (at Stage 7 above).

This base is commonly used for the preparation of pessaries, as described in Example 9.6.

Example 9.6 **Prepare 12 Pessaries Containing 10% Ichthammol.**

A 4-g mould (calibration value 4.0) is used.
Calculate for 14 pessaries to allow for wastage. Additional base is required because it is denser than the oily bases. The density factor is 1.2.

Mould calibration for glycerol-gelatin base is $4.0 \times 1.2 = 4.8$ g.

A DV is not required because the ichthammol is expressed as a percentage.

Formula for the base:

Gelatin	14 g
Glycerol	70 g
Water	to 100 g

Formula for the pessaries:

| Ichthammol | 10% w/w |
| Glycerol-gelatin base | 90% w/w |

The total weight required to prepare the pessaries is 14×4.8 g $= 67.2$ g. For ease of calculation prepare 70 g. Quantities are therefore:

| Ichthammol | 7 g |
| Base | 63 g |

Containers for suppositories

Glass or plastic screw-topped jars are the best choice of container for extemporaneously prepared suppositories and pessaries. Cardboard cartons may be used but these offer little protection from moisture or heat for hygroscopic materials.

Shelf-life

Suppositories and pessaries are relatively stable preparations, if well packaged and stored at a low temperature. Unless other information is available, an expiry date of 1 month is appropriate.

It is advisable to make a small excess of base, taking care to choose quantities which give easily weighable amounts, i.e. do not try to weigh to several decimal points. In this case 65 g can be prepared.

Using the method described previously, prepare 65 g of the base, taking care that the correct type of gelatin is chosen. Because the active ingredient is ichthammol, Type B

should be used. When the 65 g of base has been prepared, 2 g should be removed from the basin, leaving the required 63 g. The base is removed from the heat, allowed to cool a little before 7 g of ichthammol is added with careful stirring. The mixture is then poured into the lubricated mould and left to set.

Labelling for suppositories

Adequate information should appear on the label so that the patient knows how to use the product. In addition, the following information should appear: 'Store in a cool place' and 'For rectal use only' or 'For vaginal use only', whichever is appropriate.

Patient advice

In addition to what appears on the label, patients should be told to unwrap the suppository or pessary (this may appear to be unnecessary advice but there is sufficient evidence to show that it is not always done) and insert it as high as possible into the rectum or vagina. It may be helpful to provide the patient with a diagram and instruction leaflet, such as that produced by the National Pharmaceutical Association. When suppositories are for children, it is likely that an adult will have to carry out the insertion.

Key points

- Both rectal and vaginal administration can be used for local or systemic drug action
- Bases may be fatty or water miscible
- Synthetic fatty bases are easier to use than theobroma oil
- Glycerol-gelatin base produces a laxative effect
- Type A (anionic) or Type B (cationic) gelatin can be used to avoid incompatibilities
- Macrogol bases are blends of high and low molecular weight polymers which dissolve in rectal contents
- Suppository moulds have nominal capacities of 1, 2, 4 and 8 g and must be calibrated with the base to be used
- When using theobroma oil and glycerol-gelatin base, the mould has to be lubricated
- To allow for contraction on cooling, overfilling with oily bases is required
- Each mould should be calibrated for each base

- Because glycerol-gelatin base has a higher density than fatty bases, moulds hold approximately 1.2 times the nominal weight
- The displacement value (DV) is the number of parts by weight of drug which displaces one part by weight of base

- Unless the density of the drug and base are the same, a DV is required to calculate the amount of base displaced by the drug
- Labels should include either 'For rectal use only' or 'For vaginal use only', and 'Store in a cool place'

Powders and granules

Arthur J. Winfield

Introduction

A powder may be defined as a solid material in a finely divided state. Granules are powders agglomerated to produce larger free-flowing particles. Powders and granules can be used to prepare other formulations, such as solutions, suspensions and tablets. A powdered drug on its own can be a dosage form for taking orally (called a *simple powder*), when they are usually mixed with water first, or for external application as a dusting powder. Alternatively, the drug may be blended with other ingredients (called a *compound powder*).

Powders for internal use

Powders for oral administration will comprise the active ingredients with excipients such as diluents, sweeteners and dispersing agents. These may be presented as undivided powders (bulk powders) or divided powders (individually wrapped doses).

Individually wrapped powders tend not to be official formulae and are rarely prescribed these days (see Examples 10.1 and 10.2). Magnesium Trisilicate Powder Compound BP (see Example 10.4) and Compound Kaolin Powder BP are examples of bulk powders for internal use. Proprietary powders and granules include Dioralyte, Electrolade (both oral rehydration salts), Normacol (sterculia) and Fybogel (ispaghula husk).

Bulk powders

Supplying as an undivided powder is useful for non-potent, bulky drugs with a large dose, e.g. antacids, or when the dry powder is more stable than its liquid-containing counterpart. A bulk powder can be supplied to the patient although this is rarely seen nowadays because the dosage form is inconvenient to carry and there are possible inaccuracies in measuring the dose.

Individually wrapped powders

Individually wrapped powders are used to supply some potent drugs, where accuracy of dose is important. Extemporaneously produced powders are wrapped separately in paper. They are convenient dosage forms for children's doses of drugs which are not commercially available at the strength required, such as levothyroxine (thyroxine) or ibuprofen (see Example 10.2). As time progresses, more and more liquid preparations become available and so fewer powders are produced. Sealed sachets of powders are available commercially, e.g. Paramax (paracetamol and metoclopramide) and oral rehydration salts. They are mixed with water prior to taking and are useful for patients who have difficulty swallowing or where rapid absorption of the drug is required.

Granules for internal use

Some preparations are supplied to the pharmacy as granules, for reconstitution immediately before dispensing, e.g. antibiotic suspensions. This protects drugs which are susceptible to hydrolysis or other degradation in the presence of water until the time of dispensing in order to give an adequate shelf-life.

Particle size

The particle size of a powder is described using standard descriptions given in the *British Pharmacopoeia* (BP). These refer to either the standardized sieve size that they are capable of passing through in a specified time under shaking, or to the microscopically determined particle size. Thus powders for oral use would normally be a 'moderately fine' or a 'fine' powder. The former is able to pass through a sieve of nominal mesh aperture 355 μm and the latter one of 180 μm. Comminution is the process of particle size reduction. On a small scale, this can be achieved using a mortar and pestle when it is usually called *trituration*. This is a common first step in extemporaneous dispensing, after which the powder should be passed through the appropriate sieve before weighing.

Mixing the powder

Ingredients of powders should be mixed thoroughly, using the technique of 'doubling-up' (sometimes called *geometric dilution*) to ensure an even distribution. This process involves starting with the ingredient which has the smallest bulk. In Example 10.1, this is hyoscine hydrobromide. The other ingredient(s) are added progressively in approximately equal parts by volume. In this way, the amount in the mortar is approximately doubled at each addition. Mixing in between additions continues until all the ingredients are incorporated. The powder can then be packed.

Example 10.1 Prepare four powders each containing 300 μg of hyoscine hydrobromide.

Calculation and method of preparation. Calculate for five powders. Use lactose as the diluent, each powder to weigh 120 mg.
    Hyoscine hydrobromide (5 × 300)
    =1500 μg = 1.5 mg
    Lactose (5 × 120 mg) to 600 mg
    The minimum weighable quantity (using a Class B balance) is 100 mg.

Step A

Make a 1 in 10 dilution of hyoscine hydrobromide with lactose:
    Hyoscine hydrobromide 100 mg
    Lactose 900 mg
    Mix by doubling-up and remove 100 mg (triturate A).
    100 mg of triturate A contains 100/1000 × 100 = 10 mg hyoscine hydrobromide.

Example 10.1—cont'd

Step B

Make a 1 in 10 dilution of triturate A with lactose:

Triturate A	100 mg
Lactose	900 mg

Mix by doubling-up and remove 150 mg (triturate B).
    150 mg of triturate B contains 10/1000 × 150 = 1.5 mg hyoscine hydrobromide.

Step C

Triturate B	150 mg

Lactose ((5 × 120 mg) − 150 mg) = 450 mg
    Mix by doubling-up; 120-mg portions of this final powder will contain 300 μg of hyoscine hydrobromide. Weigh 120-mg aliquots and wrap in a powder paper.

Preparing individually wrapped powders

The minimum weight of an individually wrapped powder is 120 mg. Dilution of a drug with a diluent, usually lactose, is often necessary to produce this weight.

Occasionally, manufactured tablets or capsules may be used to prepare oral powders (see Example 10.2). This involves either crushing the tablet in a mortar and pestle, or emptying the contents of the capsule and adding a suitable diluent. Lactose is the most commonly used diluent because it is colourless, odourless, soluble, and has good flow properties. Some patients may be unable to tolerate lactose and suitable inert alternative diluents include light kaolin and starch.

Powder calculations

Quantities should be calculated to allow for loss of powder during manipulation. It is usual to allow for at least one extra powder. If the total amount of active ingredient required is less than the minimum weighable quantity, dilutions will be necessary. In this process, also called *trituration*, the minimum quantity of the active ingredient(s) is weighed and diluted, over several steps if necessary, in order to obtain the dose(s) required. Example 10.1 illustrates the process where two dilution steps are required.

Folding papers

White glazed paper, called *demy paper*, is used for wrapping powders. A suitable size is 120 mm × 100 mm. The wrapping should be carried out on a clean tile or larger sheet of demy

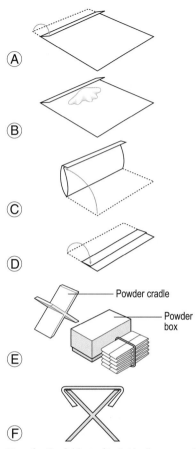

A

B

C

D

Powder cradle

Powder box

E

F

Fig. 10.1 Steps for the folding of individually wrapped powders.

to protect the product. The papers should be folded with their long edges parallel to the front of the bench. Follow the steps illustrated in Figure 10.1 in order to fold the paper:

- The long edge, furthest away from the dispenser, should be turned over to about one-seventh of the paper width (step A)
- The powder should be weighed accurately and placed on the paper towards the folded edge of the centre of the paper (step B)
- The unfolded long edge (nearest the dispenser) should then be brought over the powder to meet the crease of the folded edge and the flap closed over it (step C)
- The folded edge should then be folded over (towards the dispenser) so that it covers about half the powder packet (step D)
- The short edges of the powder packet should be folded over, using a powder cradle if available, so that the flaps are of equal lengths and the folded powder fits neatly into a box or jar (steps E and F). Before making these folds, ensure that there is no powder in the ends to be folded, otherwise it may fall out and be lost.

The creases can be sharpened with a spatula, taking care not to tear the paper or use excessive pressure which would compress the powder inside the pack.

The powders can be packed in pairs, back to back, or in one bundle, with the final powder placed back to back. They should be held together with an elastic band. In a well-wrapped product, there will be no powder in the fold or flaps, so that all the powder is available for easy administration when unwrapped.

Manufactured powders are subject to a uniformity of weight test, or uniformity of content test if each dose contains <2 mg of active ingredient or the content of active ingredient represents <2% of the total weight.

Shelf-life and storage of internal powders

Extemporaneously prepared powders should have an expiry of between 2 and 4 weeks. Proprietary powders often have a longer shelf-life because of the protective packaging. Some powders may be hygroscopic, deliquescent or volatile and will need to be protected from decomposition. Storage for these powders should be moisture proof and airtight.

Containers for internal powders

Extemporaneously prepared individually wrapped powders are often dispensed in a paperboard box. However, it is preferable to use a screw-top glass or plastic container which provides an airtight seal and protection against moisture. Proprietary powders in individual sachets which are moisture proof may be dispensed in a paperboard box. Bulk powders are packed in an airtight glass or plastic jar. A 5-mL spoon should also be supplied with bulk powders.

Special labels and advice for internal powders

Powders are usually mixed with water or another suitable liquid before taking, depending on their solubility. Powders for babies or young children can be placed directly into the mouth on the back of the tongue, followed by a drink to wash down the powder. Bulk powders should be shaken and measured carefully before dissolving or dispersing in a little water and taking.

Example 10.2 **Prepare 18 powders each containing 140 mg of ibuprofen.**

	For 1 powder	For 20 powders (2 excess)
Ibuprofen	140 mg	2.8 g

Formulation notes. A diluent is not required, since the weight of each powder will be above the minimum 120 mg required. Pure ibuprofen powder can be used. However, if it is not available, manufactured 200 mg ibuprofen tablets (not modified release) can be used to prepare these powders.

Method of preparation. Take 14 × 200 mg ibuprofen tablets (contain 2.8 g ibuprofen) and weigh them. This is necessary to allow for the weight of the tablet excipients. Grind to a fine powder in a mortar and pestle. Pass the resulting powder through a 250-μm sieve and lightly remix. Divide the original weight of tablets by 20, and weigh aliquots of the resulting amount of powder. Pack into individual powder papers. Fasten the 18 powders together with an elastic band and pack in an amber glass jar or plastic container with a screw cap.

Shelf-life and storage. Store in a cool, dry place. A shelf-life of 2–3 weeks is appropriate.

Powders for external use

Powders, with or without medicament, are frequently applied to the skin. Dusting powders contain one or more substances in fine powder and may be dispensed as single-dose or multi-dose preparations (see Example 10.3). They are used to treat a variety of skin conditions or to soothe skin. Examples are antifungal powders for athlete's foot or talc dusting powder for the prevention of chafing and skin irritation. Zinc oxide and starch are added to formulations to absorb moisture and talc is used for lubricant properties. Talc, kaolin and other natural mineral materials are liable to contamination with bacteria such as *Clostridium tetani*, *C. perfringens* and *Bacillus anthracis*. These ingredients should be sterilized by dry heat or the final product should be sterilized. Dusting powders should be sterile if they are to be applied to large areas of open skin or wounds. They should not be used where there is a likelihood of large volumes of exudate, as hard crusts will form.

Preparing powders for external use

A sieve size of 180 μm should be used to obtain the finely divided powder. The constituents should be mixed using the doubling-up method, as described previously.

Shelf-life and storage for powders for external use

Dry powders should remain stable over a long period of time if packaged and protected from the atmosphere. For extemporaneously prepared products, an expiry of 4 weeks is appropriate.

Containers for powders for external use

Powders for external use may be packed in glass, metal or plastic containers with a sifter-type cap. Some are also available commercially in pressurized containers, containing other excipients such as a propellant and lubricants.

Special labels and advice for powders for external use

'For external use only' and 'Store in a cool, dry place'.

Examples of official powders for external use include Zinc Oxide Dusting Powder Compound BPC, Chlorhexidine Dusting Powder BP and Talc Dusting Powder BP. There are now few proprietary examples of powders for external use, one being Daktarin (miconazole).

Example 10.3 **Prepare 100 g of Zinc, Starch and Talc Dusting Powder BPC.**

	Master formula	For 100 g
Zinc oxide	25%	25 g
Starch	25%	25 g
Sterilized purified talc	50%	50 g

Method of preparation. Sieve the powders, using a 180-μm sieve, weigh and mix them by doubling-up in a mortar and pestle. Pack in an amber glass jar or plastic container with a screw cap (with a perforated, reclosable lid if possible).

Shelf-life and storage. Store in a dry place. An expiry date of 4 weeks is advisable.

Example 10.4 **Prepare 200 g of Compound Magnesium Trisilicate Oral Powder BP 1988.**

	Master formula	For 200 g
Magnesium trisilicate	250 mg	50 g
Chalk	250 mg	50 g
Heavy magnesium carbonate	250 mg	50 g
Sodium bicarbonate	250 mg	50 g

Method of preparation. Sieve the powders, using a 250-μm sieve, weigh and mix them by doubling-up, using a mortar and pestle. Pack in an amber glass jar or plastic container with a screw cap.

Shelf-life and storage. Store in a dry place. A 4-week expiry date is reasonable if kept dry.

Key points

- Powders may be prepared as bulk powders, divided powders or granules
- Powders may be used internally or externally
- The particle size of a fine powder should be less than 180 μm
- The minimum weight of a divided powder is 120 mg
- Lactose is a good diluent for internal powders
- Trituration is the process used to obtain small doses which are below the minimum weighable quantity
- Ideally powders should be packed in a glass or plastic container
- A 5-mL spoon should be provided with bulk powders for oral use
- When dispensing divided powders, an excess of one or two should be prepared to allow for losses during processing

Chapter | **11** |

Production of sterile products

Derek G. Chapman

STUDY POINTS

- The requirements for sterile production
- Grades of clean areas
- Design and operation of clean areas
- Isolators
- Environmental monitoring
- Preparation of aseptic products

Introduction

The production of sterile medicinal products has special requirements. These products must be produced in conditions that ensure that they are pure. They must also be free from viable organisms and pyrogens with limited or, ideally, no particulate contamination. It is therefore important that only carefully regulated and tested procedures are used to manufacture sterile products.

Owing to their special manufacturing requirements, sterile medicines are prepared in special facilities known as *clean rooms*. These rooms are designed to reduce the risk of microbial and particulate contamination at all stages of the manufacturing process.

The clean area used to produce sterile products is commonly designed as a suite of clean rooms. With this system, the operators enter the clean rooms by way of a changing room. Within this area, the operators put on clean room clothing before entering into the clean rooms. The changing room has a lower standard of environmental quality. A clean room with a lower environmental standard is also used to prepare solutions. These solutions are then sterilized by filtration before being transferred into the filling room. The clean room used to fill and seal the product containers is the highest quality of clean room. This will reduce the risk of product contamination.

Sterile products that are marketed in the European Union must be produced in conditions, which conform with the conditions given in the revised Annex 1 of Good Manufacturing Practices (Volume IV) of *The Rules Governing Medicinal Products in the European Union*. This guidance on the procedures for manufacturing sterile products describes the cleanliness of the clean room environment and recommends how pharmaceutical clean rooms should be built and used.

Sterile product production

Production of sterile products should be carried out in a clean environment, with a limit for the environmental quality of particulate and microbial contamination. This limit for contamination is necessary to reduce the risk of product contamination. In addition, however, the temperature, humidity and air pressure of the environment should be regulated to suit the clean room processes and the comfort of the operators.

Clean areas for the production of sterile products are classified into grades A, B, C and D. These grades are categorized by the particulate quality of the environmental air when the clean area is operating in both a 'manned' and 'unmanned' state. In addition, these areas are graded by the microbial monitoring of the environmental air, surfaces and operators when the area is functioning. The standards are shown in Tables 11.1 and 11.2.

There are two common procedures used to manufacture sterile products. The first method involves the preparation of products that will be terminally sterilized. The second method involves the aseptic filling of containers

Table 11.1 Airborne particle contamination for manned and unmanned clean rooms

| | MAXIMUM NUMBER OF PARTICLES PER CUBIC METRE EQUAL TO OR ABOVE THE SIZE INDICATED | | | |
| | CLEAN ROOM AT REST | | CLEAN ROOM OPERATING | |
Grade	0.5 μm	5 μm	0.5 μm	5 μm
A	3500	1	3500	1
B	3500	1	350,000	2000
C	350,000	2000	3,500,000	20,000
D	3,500,000	20,000	Varies with procedure	Varies with procedure

Table 11.2 Limits for microbial contamination of an operating clean room

Grade	Viable organisms per cubic metre of air	90 mm settle plate per 4 h	55 mm contact plate	Glove print (5 fingers)
A	<1	<1	<1	<1
B	10	5	5	5
C	100	50	25	N/A
D	200	100	50	N/A

that are not exposed to terminal sterilization. Aseptic filling requires a higher environmental quality for the preparation of solutions, and the filling of containers. The qualities of the clean rooms used for these production procedures are detailed in Tables 11.3 and 11.4.

Premises

The sterile production unit must be separated from the general manufacturing area within the hospital pharmacy or factory. This sterile production unit must not be accessible to unauthorized personnel.

The unit is designed to allow each stage of production to be segregated. It should also ensure a safe and organized workflow, and reduce the need for personnel to move around the clean rooms. The unit is built and the equipment positioned to protect the product from contamination. The layout must allow efficient cleaning of the area and avoid the build-up of dust. Premises are also arranged to decrease the risk of mix up or contamination of one product or material by another.

The filling room is typically serviced from an adjacent preparation room. This allows supporting personnel to assemble and prepare materials. Staff within the filling room area then use these materials. Fig. 11.1 shows the layout of rooms for the production of terminally sterilized medicines, such as small or large volume injections.

Design and construction

Access to clean and aseptic filling areas is limited to authorized personnel. Operators enter clean rooms by way of changing rooms. Within the changing room, the operators can don and remove their clean room garments.

A low physical barrier, commonly known as a *pass-over* (or *cross-over*) *bench*, extends across the changing room. It forms a physical barrier that separates the different areas for changing by the operators.

Special precautions are needed to avoid contamination of clean and aseptic filling areas when materials are passed through airlocks or hatchways. Thus sterilizers and entry ports are fitted with double-sided doors. The doors are interlocked to prevent both doors being opened simultaneously.

Surfacing materials

All clean room surfaces, including the floors, walls and ceilings, should be smooth, impervious and unbroken. This will decrease the release and build-up of contaminating particles and organisms. The surfaces are made of materials that allow the use of cleaning agents and

Table 11.3 Conditions for preparing terminally sterilized products

Procedure	Required standard before terminal sterilization
Preparation of solutions for filtration and sterilization	Grade C is used for products which support microbial growth Grade D acceptable if solutions subsequently filtered
Filling small and large volume parenterals	Grade C. For products with a high risk of contamination, such as wide-necked containers, a Grade A laminar airflow workstation with Grade C background
Preparation and filling of ointments, creams, suspensions and emulsions	Grade C

Table 11.4 Conditions for the production of aseptically prepared products

Procedure	Required standard
Handling of sterile starting materials	Grade A with Grade B background, or Grade C if solution filtered later in production process
Preparation of production solutions	Grade A with Grade B background, or Grade C if sterile during filtered production
Filling of aseptically prepared products such as small and large volume parenterals	Grade A with Grade B background
Preparation and filling of ointments, creams, suspensions and emulsions	Grade A with Grade B background

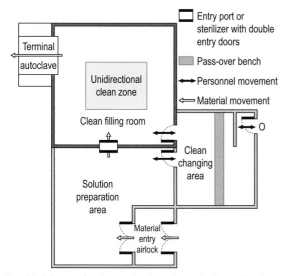

Fig. 11.1 Rooms for the production of terminally sterilized medicines.

disinfectants. The ceilings are sealed to prevent the entry of contaminants from the space above them. Unclean-able recesses within the clean room should be avoided. This will reduce the collection of contaminating particles. Thus the junction between the wall and the floor is commonly coved. The presence of shelves, ledges, cupboards and equipment is minimized. Windows should be non-opening and sealed. This will prevent the ingress of contaminants.

Services

Piped liquids and gases should be filtered before entering the clean room. This will ensure that the liquid or gas at the work position will be as clean as the clean room air. The pipes and ducts must be positioned for easy cleaning. All other fittings, such as fuse boxes and switch panels, should be positioned outside the clean rooms.

Sinks and drains must be excluded from areas where aseptic procedures are performed in clean room areas. They should be avoided in the whole unit wherever possible. In areas where sinks and drains are installed, they must be designed, positioned and maintained to decrease the risk of microbial contamination. They are thus often fitted with easily cleanable traps. The traps may contain electrically heated devices for disinfection.

There should be a limited number of entry doors for personnel and ports for materials. Entry doors should be self-closing and allow the easy movement of personnel.

Airlock doors, wall ports, through-the-wall autoclaves and dry heat sterilizers should be fitted with interlocked doors. This will prevent both doors being opened simultaneously. An alarm system should be fitted to all the doors to prevent the opening of more than one door.

Lights in clean rooms are fitted flush with the ceiling to reduce the collection of dust and avoid disturbing the air-flow pattern within the room. Similarly, equipment should be positioned in clean rooms to avoid the distribution and the collection of particles and microbial contaminants.

Environmental control

Potential sources of particles and microbial contaminants occurring within the clean room are:
- The air supply of the room
- Inflow of external air
- Production of contaminants within the room.

Each of these possible sources can be minimized as described below.

Air supply

The air supply to a Grade A, B or C clean room must be filtered to ensure the removal of particulate and microbial contamination. This is carried out by filtering the air with high-efficiency particulate air (HEPA) filters. The HEPA filter should be positioned at the inlet to the clean room or close to it. A pre-filter may be fitted upstream of the HEPA filter. This will prolong the life of the final filter. A fan is required to pump the air through the filter.

The HEPA filters use pleated fibreglass paper as the filter medium. Parallel pleats of this filter material increase the surface area of the filter and increase the airflow through the filter. This structure allows the filter to retain a compact volume. Aluminium foil is used to form spacers in the traditional type of HEPA filter. Spacers are not used in the more modern 'mini-pleat' type of filter design. These mini-pleat filters are now widely used. They have a shallower depth in construction than the traditional HEPA filter. Within the structure of the filter, the filter material is sealed to an aluminium frame (Fig. 11.2). At least one side of the filter is protected with a coated mild steel mesh. HEPA filters exhibit:
- A high flow rate
- High particulate holding capacity
- Low-pressure drop across the filter.

HEPA filters remove larger particles from the air by inertial impaction, the medium-sized particles by direct interception and the small particles by Brownian diffusion. The HEPA filters are least efficient at removing particles of about 0.3 μm. However, the efficiency of removing particles is affected by the air velocity and the filter packing. Larger and smaller particles will be removed more efficiently.

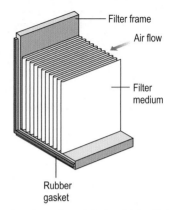

Fig. 11.2 Section through a mini-pleat high-efficiency filter, showing its construction.

With a new HEPA filter fitted in a clean room, the air exits from the filter face at a rate of about 0.45 m/s, and has a 99.997% efficiency at removing 0.3 μm particles. The pressure difference across the depth of a new filter is about 130 Pascal (Pa). At the end of the effective life of the filter, the pressure drop across the filter will increase to about 490 Pa. To retain the operating efficiency of the filter, the fan forcing air through the filter must be able to maintain this pressure difference. Sensors are fitted upstream and downstream of the filters to indicate the pressure differential across the filter. An automatic alarm system should be fitted to indicate failure in the air supply or filter blockage.

The HEPA filters for clean room use must conform with the British Standard 5295 (1989) aerosol test. The filters may have faulty seals and can be damaged during delivery or installation. It is thus important that they are tested in situ before use.

The filter material possesses a uniform resistance and is constructed with a large number of parallel pleats. This results in the air downstream of the filter face flowing uniformly with a unidirectional configuration.

The number of air changes in clean rooms is affected by:
- The room size
- The equipment in use
- The number of operators in the area.

In practice, 25–35 air changes per hour are common. The airflow pattern within the clean room must be carefully regulated to avoid generating particles from the clean room floor and from the operators. Various options for ventilating clean rooms may be categorized by the airflow pattern within the room. These are:
- Unidirectional airflow systems
- Non-unidirectional airflow systems
- Combination airflow systems.

Unidirectional airflow systems

Air enters the room through a complete wall or ceiling of high-efficiency filters. This air will sweep contamination in a single direction to the exhaust system on the opposing wall or floor (Fig. 11.3). In the interests of economy, the exhaust grill may be fitted low down on the wall. The velocity of the air is about 0.3 m/s in downflow air from ceiling filters, and 0.45 m/s in crossflow air. These are highly efficient airflow systems. However, one major disadvantage of these rooms for pharmaceutical use is that they are expensive to construct. They also use much more conditioned air than rooms with non-unidirectional airflow. This greatly increases their operating costs. Owing to these factors, unidirectional airflow clean rooms are seldom used for pharmaceutical purposes.

Non-unidirectional airflow systems

Air enters the clean rooms through filters and diffusers that are usually located in the ceiling. It exits through outlet ducts positioned low down on the wall or in the floor, at sites remote from the air inlet (Fig. 11.4). With the use of this system, the filtered inlet air mixes with, and dilutes, the contaminated air within the room. As the clean room air has been previously heated and cleaned, it can be recirculated to save energy, a little fresh air being introduced with each air change cycle.

Various designs of diffuser are used with this ventilation system. These affect the air movement and the cleanliness of the rooms. The perforated plate diffuser produces a jet flow of air directly beneath it. This jet of air will carry contamination at its edges. However, it does produce high-quality air directly under the diffuser. It is thus important that production procedures are located directly below the diffuser. By contrast, the air released from the bladed diffuser will mix with the clean room air. This diffuser thus produces a reasonably constant quality of air throughout the room.

Combination systems

In many pharmaceutical clean rooms, it is common to find that the background area is ventilated by a non-unidirectional airflow system. Meanwhile, the critical areas are supplied with high-quality air from unidirectional airflow units.

The combination airflow system is often selected for pharmaceutical clean room applications as it:
- Produces controlled room pressure
- Separates the manufacturing process from the general clean room
- Is cheaper to use.

Several types of unidirectional flow workstations or benches are used in this combination-type room. Various

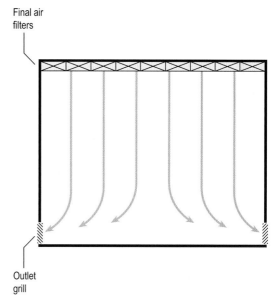

Fig. 11.3 Airflow pattern in a unidirectional airflow clean room.

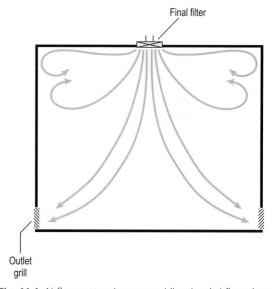

Fig. 11.4 Airflow pattern in a non-unidirectional airflow clean room.

vertical unidirectional airflow systems are used in combination clean rooms. With one system, the critical area is surrounded by a plastic curtain with vertical unidirectional downflow air 'washing' over the manufacturing process, and exiting under the plastic curtains into the general clean

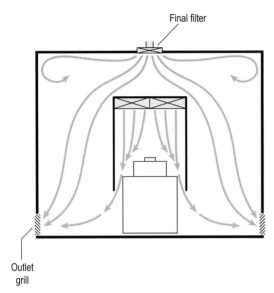

Fig. 11.5 Airflow patterns in a mixed-flow clean room with non-unidirectional airflow background environment, and unidirectional airflow protection for a critical area.

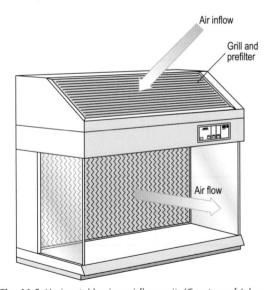

Fig. 11.6 Horizontal laminar airflow unit. (Courtesy of John Bass Ltd.)

room area (Fig. 11.5). An alternative system is often used with the small-scale combination-type clean room in hospital pharmacies. With this system, a horizontal airflow cabinet (Fig. 11.6) is used as the workstation. With these cabinets, a fan forces air through a HEPA filter located at the rear wall of the workstation. The air that exits from the filter first washes over the critical work area before washing over the arms and upper body areas of the operator. Contamination arising from the operator is thus kept downstream of the critical procedures. Grade A environmental conditions are achieved at the critical work area. A similar workstation known as a *vertical laminar airflow cabinet* (Fig. 11.7) could also be used in the combination room. This cabinet passes air vertically downwards from the ceiling of the cabinet over the critical working area. It produces a Grade A environmental quality. The air exits from the front of the workstation.

In recent times, there has been a trend towards protecting the critical procedures within combination clean rooms by using isolator cabinets. The isolator cabinet gives a localized high-quality environment. Isolators give protection from potential contamination in clean rooms as they are positively pressurized with air supplied through HEPA filters. The operator works outside the confines of the isolator, using glove ports, to perform procedures within the enclosed chamber. The gloved hands of clean room operators can transfer microbial contamination into critical working areas within the clean room. To indicate that the required clean room standards have been achieved (Table 11.2), the fingertips of a gloved hand are depressed onto the surface of a suitable solid growth medium. This medium is incubated to show any contamination.

There is also a need to avoid contaminated external air passing into the clean room environment. Thus the clean room air pressure must exceed that of the surrounding areas. The pressure differential between different standards of clean room should be 10–15 Pa. This level should be comparatively easy to monitor, and will decrease the unregulated outflow of air. Adjusting grills, known as *pressure stabilizers* located in the walls of rooms, regulate the outflow of clean room air and the room pressure. The air moves from an area of high pressure to an area of lower pressure. To maintain the room pressure, it is important that the rooms are airtight. However, a small quantity of air will exit from the rooms by way of door spaces.

Temperature and humidity control

The temperature and the humidity are adjusted to suit the procedures being carried out within the clean room, and maintain the comfort of the operators. A target temperature of about 20°C, with a relative humidity of about 35–45%, is usually preferred.

Personnel

The clean room environment is supplied with high-quality air at positive pressure. The main source of contamination in these areas arises from skin scales that are released by the clean room operators.

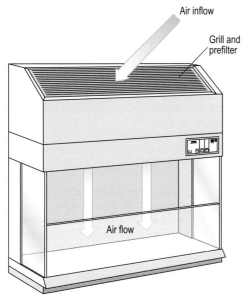

Air inflow

Grill and prefilter

Air flow

Fig. 11.7 Vertical laminar airflow unit. (Courtesy of John Bass Ltd.)

To limit clean room contamination by personnel, there is a need to:

- Restrict the number of operators working in the clean room
- Restrict operator conversations
- Instruct operators to move slowly
- Minimize general movement throughout the room
- Avoid operators interrupting the airflow between the inlet filter and the work area.

The clean room operator is constantly shedding dead skin scales from the body surface. Not all of these skin particles are contaminated with bacteria. Males shed more particles that are contaminated with bacteria than females. In addition, individual males and females show variable rates of bacterial dispersal. This dispersal from the individual is affected by:

- Personal characteristics
- General health and skin condition.

Body movements of personnel will increase the number of contaminated particles released from the skin surface. Each individual releases more than 10^6 skin scales/min during normal walking movements. There is a need to contain the dispersion of skin particles from the operators in clean rooms, and protect both the environment and the product. Containment of particles is achieved by the operators wearing clean room clothing. This clothing is made from synthetic fabrics that filter out particulate and microbial contamination from the operators, without the fabrics releasing contamination. However, this clothing is not absolute and

particles can pass through the garments. Operators wearing clean room undergarments reduce this effect. The outer garments are close fitting at the neck, wrists and ankles, but these sites still provide an exit route for particulate matter.

Clean garments should be used for each work session and must provide operator comfort. Disposable single-use garments are available, although most production units employ reusable garments. The clothing is specially laundered in an area with similar standards to those used in the clean room. Garments are laundered by a wet-wash process using particle-free solutions. This is followed by an antibacterial rinse and hot air drying, and then the garments are packaged in sealed bags to avoid particulate contamination. This cleaning process fulfils the needs of most pharmaceutical clean room applications, which are a balance between cost and acceptability. For a higher level of sterility assurance, the garments are gamma irradiated using ^{60}Co, each garment receiving an approved dose of 25 kGy. This treatment is expensive and decreases the life of the garments. The donning of clean room clothing, without contaminating the outer surface of the garments, is a rather difficult procedure that is performed in the changing room.

Changing room

Entry of personnel into clean rooms should be through a changing room fitted with interlocking doors. These doors act as an airlock to prevent the influx of external air. This access route is intended for the entry of personnel only. The changing room is subdivided into three areas. Movement through these areas must comply with a strict protocol. They are often colour coded as black, grey and white, with black representing the dirtiest area, while white represents the cleanest area.

The black area is where jewellery, cosmetics, factory or hospital protective garments, and shoes are removed. Long hair may be contained and a mobcap donned to contain the hair completely. The pass-over bench forms a physical separation between the black and the grey areas in the changing room. The operator sits on the pass-over bench, swings his/her legs over the bench and fits clean room covers over the feet before they are placed on the floor of the grey area.

The operator then stands up in the grey area. Wrappings on the various garments are opened to avoid contacting the outer surface of the packaging following the hand-washing procedure. Then the operator washes hands and forearms using an antiseptic solution. Special attention is paid to cleaning the fingernails. The hands are then dried using an automatic air-blow drier, as towels shed particles when used for drying hands.

Clothing garments are donned in sequence from head to foot. Throughout this procedure, care must be taken to avoid the hands contacting the outer surface of the clean

Table 11.5 Clothing for clean room use

Clean room grade	Description of clothing
A/B	Head cover and face mask
	Single- or two-piece trouser suit
	Overboots and sterile powder-free rubber or plastic gloves
C	Hair (and beard) cover
	Single- or two-piece trouser suit
	Clean room shoes or overshoes
D	Hair (and beard) cover
	Protective suit
	Appropriate shoes or overshoes

room clothing. First, the head and shoulder hood is fitted, ensuring that all the hair is contained within the head cover. A face mask is fitted to prevent the shedding of droplets. The one-piece coverall (or alternatively two-piece trouser suit) is put on. Care must be taken to avoid these garments contacting the floor surface. The shoulder cover of the head and shoulder hood is tucked into the coverall. Then the zip is closed and the studs fastened. Overboots are then fitted over the clean room shoes. The overboots are kept in position with ties that are suitably fastened for operator comfort. For entry into aseptic filling rooms, an antiseptic cream is applied to the hands. The clean room powder-free gloves are then donned. Care is needed to avoid contacting the outer surface of the gloves. The cuffs of the coverall are secured within the gloves and the gloved hands disinfected. The operator now enters into the white clean room area, and begins work. During the work procedures, the gloved hands of the operators are regularly disinfected. Key features of the clothing are given in Table 11.5.

Cleaning

A strict cleaning and disinfection policy is essential to minimize particulate and microbial contamination in the clean room. Operators release microbial and particulate contamination within the clean room. These contaminants are mostly deposited onto horizontal surfaces. However, other areas of the clean room can become contaminated due to direct contact with the operators' clothing. It is thus essential that a strict cleaning and disinfection policy is implemented within the clean room to minimize both the particulate, and the microbial contamination.

There are two main methods of cleaning. Vacuuming is effective at removing gross particulate contamination of particles greater than 100 μm. However, vacuuming is not very effective at removing smaller particles. Small particles are removed by wet wiping. It is important that the wet wipe is sterile, and must not generate particulate contamination. The use of wet wipes involves the use of cleaning agents that will remove particulate contamination and have an antibacterial effect.

The ideal cleaning agent should be:
- Effective in removing undesirable contamination
- Harmless to surfaces
- Fast drying
- Non-flammable
- Non-toxic
- Cost-effective.

Anionic or cationic surfactants are used as cleaning agents within the clean room. The disinfectants of choice for clean room use are generally quaternary ammonium compounds, phenols, alcohols and polymeric biguanides. The disinfectant solutions should be freshly prepared before use. Different types of disinfectants should be used in rotation to prevent the development of resistant microbial strains. Most surfactants or detergents will dissipate surface static electricity, but the most effective and widely used antistatic agents used in clean rooms are cationic surfactants.

Trained personnel regularly clean critical production areas of clean rooms. A less stringent cleaning protocol is required in the general clean room areas. This applies to the walls and floors where contamination cannot directly contaminate the product. As part of the cleaning protocol, regular microbiological monitoring should be carried out to determine the effectiveness of the disinfection procedures.

Isolators

Commercial manufacturers are using isolators increasingly for the aseptic filling of products, with combination isolators being used. Isolators are also used for sterility testing of products. Robots have been used in isolators for repetitive processes, such as sterility testing, but they are expensive. Isolators are used in hospital pharmacy departments, as an alternative to clean rooms, for the small-scale aseptic processing of sterile products. Aseptic procedures performed in the best isolators cannot reach the same levels of sterility assurance achieved by terminal heat sterilization (see Table 11.6). However, when suitably operated, they can produce a sterility assurance level better than the conventional clean room. Isolators are often selected for aseptic manipulations of sterile products as they are:
- Relatively inexpensive
- Easily designed for a specific purpose
- Capable of providing operator protection from the product.

Table 11.6 Microbial contamination of batch-produced sterile products

Place of production	Microbial contamination
Industrial production	
Terminal sterilization by dry or moist heat or irradiation	1 in at least 10^6 containers
Aseptic preparation in sealed gassed isolator using sophisticated transfer system	1 in 10^6
Aseptic preparation in conventional clean room using sophisticated laminar airflow system	1 in 10^5
Aseptic preparation in conventional clean room	1 in 10^4
Aseptic complex preparation of large-volume total parenteral nutrition fluids	1 in 10^3
Production in hospital pharmacy	
Terminal sterilization by dry or moist heat containers	1 in at least 10^6
Aseptic preparation in an isolator with surfaces cleaned and wiped with sterile alcohol. Extensively used in many pharmacies	1 in 10^3
Aseptic preparation in a well-managed clean room	1 in 10^3 (or less)

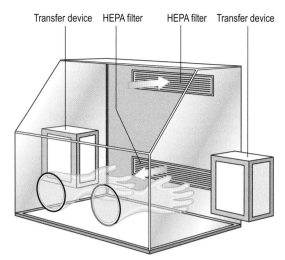

Fig. 11.8 Isolator cabinet.

Isolators are composed of a chamber that controls the environment surrounding the work procedure (Fig. 11.8). The inlet and exhaust air passes through HEPA filters. The airflow pattern within the isolator chamber may be either unidirectional, non-unidirectional, or a combination of both. Vertical unidirectional airflow has the advantage of rapidly purging particles from the isolator chamber. This is an advantage for aseptic processes. The air within the isolator chamber should be frequently changed to maintain the aseptic chamber environment. Particle and microbial contamination of the environment within the isolator chamber must conform with the Grade A standard as detailed in Tables 11.1 and 11.2.

The operator remains outside the isolator chamber environment. To perform manual manipulations within the chamber, the operator inserts his hands and arms into the chamber. Entry occurs by way of a glove port, using either a one-piece full-arm-length glove or a glove and sleeve system. With the glove and sleeve system, the easily changeable glove is attached to a sleeve that is attached to the wall of the chamber through an airtight seal. Using either of these glove systems, the operator is able to perform aseptic manipulations in comfort, up to a distance of about 0.5 m within the chamber. The glove system avoids contamination arising from the operator, and maintains the integrity of the isolator chamber environment. As cytotoxic materials can diffuse through the gloves, it is important that they are changed regularly. To perform the work procedure within the chamber, materials must be introduced and prepared products removed without compromising the chamber environment. This transfer procedure is a critical factor in the operation of the isolator and is carried out using a transfer system. The transfer system separates the external environment from the controlled isolator environment. It restricts airflow between these areas, while allowing the transfer of materials between them. The transfer system is fitted with an interlocked double door entry system. This will provide an airlock that avoids both doors being opened to the external environment simultaneously. A filtered air inlet and exhaust is fitted to the transfer system. However, a risk of microbial contamination during the transfer does exist. The isolator must be positioned in a suitable background environment of at least a Grade D classification. This is typically achieved by positioning the isolator in a dedicated room that is only used for the isolator and its related activities.

Isolators are divided into positive and negative pressure isolators.

Positive pressure isolator

This isolator operates under positive pressure, and protects the product from contamination arising from an external source and from the aseptic process itself. It is used for the aseptic preparation of pharmaceutical products and can be used as a sterility test chamber.

Negative pressure isolator

This isolator will protect the product from contamination arising from an external source, and from the aseptic manipulation. In addition, however, this isolator should protect the operator from hazardous materials, such as cytotoxic preparations or radiopharmaceuticals, in the isolator chamber. This type of isolator operates under negative pressure. The exhaust air is ducted to the outside through at least one HEPA filter, and through an adsorption material, such as activated carbon. Rigid negative pressure isolators should be used for radiopharmaceutical manipulations. In this situation, the isolator is frequently used with a lead-free vision panel, and a lead glass protector around the product. Alternatively, isolators are available with lead acrylic glass windows.

The chambers of isolators are gas sterilized. The ideal sterilant for use in the isolator chamber should have the following properties:
- Non-corrosive to metals and plastics
- Rapidly lethal to all microorganisms
- Good penetration
- Harmless.

The sterilants in most general use for pharmaceutical applications in isolators do not comply with all of these ideal properties. Those used are peracetic acid vapour and hydrogen peroxide vapour. To reduce the risk of chemical contamination of the sterile product, the sterilant contact time should be carefully regulated. The sterilant must be flushed from the isolator before beginning the aseptic manipulations.

Currently marketed isolators are constructed with either a flexible canopy, or a rigid containment medium. The rigid type of isolator is often preferred, owing to the reduced risk of the chamber being punctured. This occurs more readily with the flexible canopy design. Rigid isolators are often constructed from a stainless-steel frame with a moulded acrylic window. A further isolator, known as a *half-suit isolator*, is currently in use. This is a flexible canopy isolator that is made from material such as nylon-lined polyvinyl chloride. It is designed using a half-suit sealed to a wall of the chamber. This system allows the torso of the operator to be introduced into the suit that is located within the chamber of the isolator. To improve visibility, a transparent helmet is sealed to the neck of the suit that is ventilated by a pressurized air supply. This provides operator comfort over prolonged work sessions. The advantage of the half-suit isolator is that the operator can easily access a large area of the chamber, and manoeuvre heavier and larger materials. The half-suit isolator is used as dedicated production equipment for the aseptic compounding of products such as total parenteral nutrition (TPN) fluids.

During a 2-week period in September 1992, eight children died from infection after receiving contaminated TPN fluids at four different hospitals in South Africa. These fluids had been prepared in flexible film isolators. The investigation of this incident revealed that the production equipment was suitable for its purpose but inadequate procedures had allowed contamination and subsequent growth of pathogenic bacteria in the TPN fluids. It should therefore be carefully noted that the use of isolators requires trained staff and good manufacturing practices to maintain product quality.

Isolator tests

Isolators must be frequently tested to ensure that they operate as a sealed chamber, and conform with the required level of air quality and surface contamination. They are thus subjected to both physical and microbial tests.

Physical tests include:
- *Integrity tests.* These tests will detect leaks that compromise the integrity of the isolator chamber. The procedure is routinely carried out by sealing the chamber and recording changes in the chamber pressure over time
- *Glove inspection.* The glove and sleeve are visually inspected and leak tested for pin holes
- *HEPA filter test.* The integrity of the HEPA filter should be tested with an aerosol generator and a detector
- *Airborne particle count.* This is carried out in the isolator chamber and the transfer device using a particle counter.

Microbial tests use microbial growth media suitable for the growth of potential contaminants. The tests include:
- *Active air sampling.* This test determines the number of organisms in the air of the isolator chamber. The procedure uses impact and agar impingement samplers
- *Settle plates.* Settle plates containing growth media are exposed in the chamber for 2–4 h. Particles and organisms settle by gravity onto the agar surface. The plates are then incubated
- *Surface tests.* Surfaces are sampled using direct contact plates that are then incubated. Following sampling, it is important to remove materials deposited onto the sampled surfaces during the test. Alternatively, surfaces are sampled using sterile moistened swabs. The swabs are then streaked onto solid growth media, and incubated. Soluble swabs may be dissolved in sterile diluent, and the viable count determined
- *Finger dabs.* The fingertips of the gloved hand are pressed onto the surface of solid growth medium. The medium is then incubated
- *Broth fill test.* This test challenges both the manipulative procedure of the operator and the facilities. The test simulates routine aseptic procedures by using nutrient medium in place of a product to produce broth-filled units. These units are incubated to indicate microbial contamination.

Environmental monitoring

Following construction of a clean room, it must be tested to ensure that it is providing the required quality of environment. These verification tests are rigorously performed and are similar to the tests that are used to monitor the clean room. The monitoring tests ensure that the clean room continues to provide satisfactory operation.

To ensure that the pharmaceutical clean room is providing the required environmental standards, the following are determined.

Air quality

The air supplied to the clean room must not contribute to particulate or microbial contamination within the room. The HEPA filters for the inlet air must be tested to ensure that neither the filter fabric nor the filter seals are leaking. This is done by introducing a smoke with a known particle size upstream of the filter. The clean room surface of the filter is then scanned for smoke penetration using a photometer or a particle counter.

Air movement

Adequate ventilation throughout the clean room can be determined by air movement tests. These are carried out at the time of clean room validation. Air movement within the clean room is determined by measuring the decay profile of smoke particles released into the clean room. Smoke particle release is also used to ensure that a clean area within a unidirectional workstation is not being contaminated with air from the clean room environment.

The outflow of air from a clean room, with a higher standard of cleanliness, to an area with a lower standard is indicated by the pressure differential between the rooms. This is determined using a manometer or magnehelic gauge.

Air velocity

The velocity of the air at several points in a clean room area of critical importance should be determined. This is done both at validation of the clean room and at timed intervals. The procedure involves the use of an anemometer.

Airborne particulate and microbial contamination

The particle count, and the microbial bioburden of the clean room, provide the basis for the air classification system for grading a clean room, as detailed in Table 11.1. The points for sampling, and the number of samples taken at each position, are determined by the size and the grade of the clean room. Airborne particles are normally sized and counted by optical particle counters.

Microbial monitoring

There should be very few viable organisms present in the clean room air. However, operators within the clean room disperse large numbers of skin particles. Many of these particles are contaminated with bacteria. The dispersal of contaminated particles by the clean room operator is greatly decreased by the wearing of occlusive clothing, together with appropriate air ventilation. Sampling for microbial contamination is necessary when people are present in the clean room during production. Monitoring of the microbial contamination during production will ensure that both the use of clean room clothing by the operators and the air ventilation system are producing the required environmental standards. Air sampling is carried out by volumetric sampling, or by the use of settle plates. With volumetric sampling, a measured volume of air is drawn from the environment, and contaminants are impinged onto a suitable microbial growth medium. The medium is then incubated and the colonies of microbial growth counted. Settle plates rely on bacteria-carrying particles being deposited onto the exposed solid surface of sterile microbial growth media contained in a 90- or 140-mm diameter Petri dish. When positioning the plates, care is needed to avoid accidental contamination. Owing to the small number of microbial contaminants in the clean room, the settle plates are preferably exposed for about 4 h.

The surfaces of the clean room should also be tested for microbial contamination, notably in areas that may be contacted by the clothing of the operators. This is achieved by using contact plates, or by using sterile moistened swabs. The contact plates allow a sterile agar surface to be pressed onto the clean room surface. These plates are then incubated to reveal microbial growth. Swabbing procedures are carried out as previously detailed in isolator tests.

Aseptic preparation

Parenteral products such as injections, infusions and eye products must be sterile for administration to the patient (see Chs 12 and 13). The preferred method of manufacturing parenteral medicines is to place the product in its final container and then seal this package. The product is then protected from further contamination and is terminally sterilized. At worst, this achieves the risk of one product in a million being contaminated following terminal sterilization by dry or moist heat, or by irradiation. Some products cannot withstand this sterilization process. An alternative approach, known as *aseptic preparation*, must then be used to prepare these medicines. This procedure is carried out in industry with selected products, but is extensively used in hospital pharmacy where products are specially compounded to meet the specific needs of patients (see Chs 15 and 17).

As shown in Table 11.6, aseptic preparation of parenteral products provides the lowest level of assurance of sterility of all the methods currently used to produce these formulations. In the pharmaceutical industry, pre-sterilized medicines are aseptically filled into sterile containers. The filling process must avoid recontamination of the sterile medicine and its container during this process. A sterility assurance level of 10^{-6} is achieved, but to achieve this requires highly sophisticated industrial production procedures. In hospital pharmacy, pre-sterilized product components are aseptically compounded using sterile apparatus, and then aseptically added to appropriate packaging for subsequent patient administration. It is critical that the sterile product components and the packaging are not recontaminated with organisms or particulate matter during these aseptic procedures. In order to achieve this, the sterile product components and the sterile package must be manipulated in a high-quality environment. The aseptic preparation and filling of products is performed in a localized Grade A zone that is achieved by a laminar airflow cabinet with a Grade B background. The Grade A environment within an isolator cabinet is also suitable for the compounding of aseptic preparations. It is important that this quality environment is continuous throughout the aseptic preparation process. Great reliance is not only placed on the facility and equipment used to produce the product, but also on the ability of the trained operators to avoid product contamination. It achieves a sterility assurance level of about one in a thousand. The manufacture of aseptic products also needs a stringent quality assurance system to ensure production of a quality product that is fit for its intended purpose. The quality assurance system should have documented, validated and audited procedures with in-process monitoring and standard operating procedures defining each step of the production process.

There is a need for awareness of the potential risk of infection that can occur during the aseptic preparation of pharmacy products. This has been shown by the tragic outcome of the supply of contaminated parenteral nutrition fluids to children at the Royal Manchester Children's Hospital in 1994. These fluids were aseptically compounded in an isolator. Microorganisms were unknowingly transferred from a sink into the isolator chamber on components used to prepare the feeds. The contaminating organisms grew in fluid remaining in assembled tubing used to prepare the feeds in the isolator. Reuse of this tubing resulted in contamination of the feeds that infected the patients. During these events, it was shown that the equipment was not faulty, only the manner in which it had been used. This demonstrates the importance of adequately disinfecting the components being transferred into the isolator, and for a total quality system for the manufacture of aseptic products.

In order to aseptically prepare a parenteral medicine, it is critical that validated procedures are stringently followed. This must go hand in hand with the other components of the quality assurance system for the preparation of aseptically prepared products of quality that are right first time and every time.

Testing for sterility

Sterility testing is the final method of assuring sterility of the manufactured product. The test is required in most countries for assuring the sterility of aseptically prepared sterile products. Aseptic manufacturing units in hospital pharmacy often perform the test retrospectively, following patient administration. A few commercial manufacturers are exempt from performing the sterility test on products that have been terminally sterilized and prepared using highly developed quality assurance procedures, incorporating validated and controlled sterilization procedures. This has been referred to as *parametric release*.

Sterility testing attempts to indicate the presence or absence of viable microorganisms in containers selected from a batch of product. A decision is made as to the sterility of the entire batch from the results obtained by testing the sample. The test has both technical and numerical limitations, and thus only provides a partial indication to the state of sterility of each product within a manufactured batch. The numerical limitation arises as only 10% of a batch of parenteral product is sampled, but the probability of accidental contamination in an aseptically manufactured batch can be as high as one in a thousand (10^{-3}), while the probability of contamination of a terminally sterilized batch is at worst only one in a million (10^{-6}).

The details of the test for sterility are provided in the *British Pharmacopoeia* (BP 2012), and this test conforms with the standards of the *European Pharmacopoeia* (EP 2013). These are also very similar to the test in the *Japanese Pharmacopoeia* (2012) and *United States Pharmacopoeia 36* (USP 2013).

Key points

- Particulate and microbial contamination of sterile products is minimized by preparation in a clean environment
- Quality of clean areas is graded A, B, C, D in decreasing stringency for particulate and microbial content

- Premises must allow segregation of stages of production and protect products from contamination by all possible means of design and operation
- Access to clean areas is restricted, and special clothing must be worn
- Environmental control, particularly of the air supply to the room, is required to ensure a minimal contamination hazard
- HEPA filters have a 99.997% efficiency at removing 0.3µm particles, the size at which their efficiency is lowest
- Airflow may be designed as unidirectional, non-unidirectional or as a combination system
- In addition to general air quality, localized areas of higher quality can be produced either by airflow design in enclosed areas or by isolator cabinets
- The main source of contamination in clean rooms is the skin scales from operators
- Clean room clothing, made from synthetic fabrics, is designed to minimize release of operator contaminants
- Changing areas are designed and used to minimize the entry of contamination on personnel
- During cleaning, vacuuming and wet wiping are used to remove large and small particles, respectively
- Isolators give protection to both the product and the operator at relatively low cost
- Type II isolators protect the operator from hazardous materials in addition to providing the Type I facilities of protection of the product from contamination
- Isolator interiors are sterilized using a gas sterilant
- Isolator integrity is tested using physical and microbial tests
- A range of environmental tests is used in clean rooms to monitor air quality, movement and velocity, airborne particles and microbial contamination
- Aseptic preparation is involved with repackaging sterile products for patient use without terminal sterilization
- Aseptic preparation is performed in laminar airflow cabinets in clean rooms, or in isolator cabinets to avoid product contamination
- A stringent quality assurance system is required for aseptic production to ensure a quality product is prepared
- The test for sterility has numerical limitations due to the sample size – cannot guarantee to detect small levels of product contamination

Chapter | **12** |

Parenteral products

Derek G. Chapman

STUDY POINTS

- Reasons for parenteral administration
- Routes available for parenteral administration
- Forms and types of parenteral product
- Design of containers for the administration of parenteral products
- Formulation and uses of parenteral products

Introduction

In practice, parenteral products are often regarded as dosage forms that are implanted, injected or infused directly into vessels, tissues, tissue spaces or body compartments. Parenteral products are often used for drugs that cannot be given orally. This may be because of patient intolerance, the instability of the drug or poor absorption of the drug if given by the oral route. From the site of administration, the drug is transported to the site of action. With developing technology, parenteral therapy is being used outside the hospital or clinic environment: at a patient's home or their workplace, allowing self-administration.

Parenteral therapy is used to:
- Produce a localized effect
- Administer drugs if the oral route cannot be used
- Deliver drugs to the unconscious patient
- Rapidly correct fluid and electrolyte imbalances
- Ensure delivery of the drug to the target tissues.

Parenteral injections are either administered directly into blood for a fast and controlled effect, or into tissues outside the blood vessels for a local or systemic effect. An intravenously administered (IV) injection will rapidly increase the concentration of drug in the blood plasma, but this concentration falls due to the reversible transfer of the drug from blood plasma into body tissues, a process known as *distribution*. An IV infusion administers a large volume of fluid at a slow rate, and ensures that the drug enters the general circulation at a constant rate. A steady state is reached when the rate of drug addition equals the rate of drug loss in the blood plasma. When infusion is stopped, elimination of the drug from the body generally follows first-order kinetics.

Following subcutaneous (SC) and intramuscular (IM) injection, there is a delay in the systemic effects of the drug due to the time taken for the drug to first pass through the walls of the capillaries before entering into the blood. This occurs by passive diffusion that is promoted by the concentration gradient across the capillary wall. The drug concentration in the blood plasma rises to a peak level and then falls due to distribution to the tissues, followed by metabolism and excretion.

Administration procedures

IV injections and infusions

The vein that is selected for administering the formulation depends on the size of the delivery needle or catheter, the type and volume of fluid to be administered, and the rate at which the fluid is to be administered. The fluids are administered into a superficial vein, commonly on the back of the hand or in the internal flexure of the elbow. The intravenous route is widely used to administer parenteral products, but it must not be used to administer water-in-oil emulsions or suspensions.

SC injections

These are injected into the loose connective and adipose tissue immediately beneath the skin in the abdomen, the

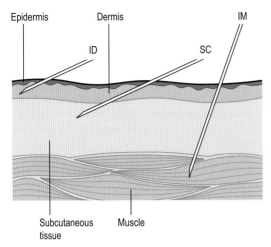

Fig. 12.1 Injection routes. *ID*, Intradermal; *IM*, intramuscular; *SC*, subcutaneous.

upper back, the upper arms and the lateral upper hips (Fig. 12.1). Typically, the volume injected does not exceed 1 mL. Following administration, the site of the injection, the body temperature, the age of the patient and the degree of massaging of the injection site will all affect the drug distribution.

IM injections

Small-volume aqueous solutions, solutions in oil and suspensions are administered directly into the body of a relaxed muscle, such as the gluteal muscle in the buttock, the deltoid muscle in the shoulder or the vastus lateralis of the thigh (Fig. 12.1).

Other routes of parenteral administration include intradermal, intra-arterial, intracardiac, intraspinal and intra-articular.

Products for parenteral use

Parenteral products include injection, infusion and implantation.

Injections

These are subdivided into small- and large-volume parenteral fluids. Small-volume parenteral fluids are sterile, pyrogen-free injectable products. They are packaged in volumes up to 100 mL. Small-volume parenteral fluids are packed as:

- Single-dose ampoules
- Multiple-dose vials
- Prefilled syringes.

Single-dose ampoules

Most small-volume parenteral fluids are currently packaged as either ampoules or vials. Glass ampoules are thin-walled containers made of Type I borosilicate glass (see Fig. 4.2). Injections packaged in glass ampoules are manufactured by filling the product into the ampoules, which are then heat sealed. To achieve the quality required of these products, the packaged solution must be sterile and practically free of particles. These products are prepared in clean room conditions (see Ch. 11). Opening glass ampoules may contaminate the product with glass particles; this is a hazard to the patient. Modern glass ampoules have weakened necks to reduce the number of particles.

Plastic ampoules are prepared, filled and sealed by a procedure known as *blow-fill-seal* in which the semi-solid plastic is blow moulded and formed into ampoules. These containers are filled with the product and immediately sealed. This system is only used to package simple solutions due to absorption of the drug by the plastic. When the ampoule is opened, only a few particles are released into the solution.

Ampoules should have a reliable seal that can be readily leak tested and will not deteriorate during the lifetime of the product. Ampoules do not contain added antimicrobial preservatives. The ampoule must contain a slight excess volume of product. This is necessary to allow the nominal injection volume to be drawn into a syringe.

Multiple-dose vials

These are composed of a thick-walled glass container that is sealed with a rubber closure. The closure is kept in position by an aluminium seal (see Fig. 4.4), then covered with a plastic cap. The cap is removed before a needle, attached to a syringe, is inserted through the rubber closure to withdraw a dose of product. The contents of the vial may be removed in several portions.

There are disadvantages with the use of glass vials. Fragments of the closure may be released into the product when the needle is inserted through the closure. There is also the risk of interaction between the product and the closure. Repeated withdrawal of injection solution from these containers increases the risk of microbial contamination of the product. These products must, therefore contain an antimicrobial preservative unless the medicine itself has antimicrobial activity. An example of such a multidose product is insulin.

Prefilled syringes

With these devices, the injection solution is aseptically filled into sterile syringes. The packed solution has a high level of sterility assurance and does not contain an antimicrobial

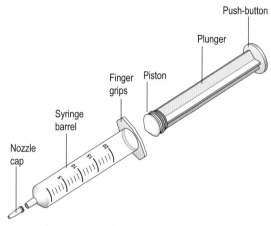

Fig. 12.2 Hypodermic syringe for single use.

preservative. The final product is available for immediate use. Prefilled syringes are becoming increasingly common.

Administration of small-volume parenteral products

Hypodermic syringes and needles are extensively used for administering small volumes of parenteral formulations to the patient. These syringes have been sterilized by ethylene oxide gas or by gamma irradiation following packaging. Various sizes of hypodermic syringes are available. They are composed of a barrel, having a graduated scale, together with a plunger and a headpiece, known as a *piston* (Fig. 12.2). These components are often made of polypropylene.

Formulation of parenteral products

Vehicles for injections

The vehicle provides the highest proportion of the formulation, and should not be toxic nor have any therapeutic activity.

Water for Injections

Water for Injections is the most extensively used vehicle in parenteral formulations. Water for Injections must be free of pyrogens and have a high level of chemical purity. The BP considers that Water for Injections can only be prepared by distillation.

Sterilized Water for Injections

This is prepared by packing a volume of Water for Injections in sealed containers. These containers are then moist-heat sterilized, which yields a sterile product that remains free of pyrogens.

Pyrogens

Pyrogens are fever-producing substances. Water is the greatest source of pyrogens in parenteral products. Pyrogens can be removed in the preparation of Water for Injections by distillation. Water that is free from pyrogens is termed *apyrogenic*.

Microbial pyrogens arise from components of Gram-negative and Gram-positive bacteria, fungi and viruses. Non-microbial pyrogens are, for example, some steroids and plasma components.

Parenteral products must be prepared in conditions that reduce microbial contamination because bacteria contaminating aqueous solutions can release pyrogens. Contaminated solutions will become more pyrogenic with the passage of time. Therefore these products must be sterilized shortly after preparation.

Dry heat at 250°C for 30 min is the most common method of inactivating pyrogens.

Non-aqueous solvents

Water-miscible co-solvents, such as glycerin and propylene glycol, are used as vehicles in small-volume parenteral fluids. They are used to increase the solubility of drugs and to stabilize drugs degraded by hydrolysis.

Metabolizable oils are used to dissolve drugs that are insoluble in water. For example, steroids, hormones and vitamins are dissolved in vegetable oils. These formulations are administered by intramuscular injection.

Additives

Various additives, such as antimicrobial agents, antioxidants, buffers, chelating agents and tonicity-adjusting agents, are included in injection formulations. Their purpose is to produce a safe and elegant product. Both the types and amounts of additives to be included in formulations are given in the appropriate monograph in the BP.

Antimicrobial agents

Antimicrobial agents are added to inhibit the growth of microbial organisms that may accidentally contaminate the product during use, for example in multiple-dose vials. The antimicrobial agents must be stable and effective in the parenteral formulation. Rubber closures have been shown to take up antimicrobial preservatives from the injection solution. Preservative uptake is more significant with natural and neoprene rubber and much less significant with butyl rubber closures.

Antioxidants

Many drugs in aqueous solutions are easily degraded by oxidation. Small-volume parenteral products of these drugs often contain an antioxidant. Bisulphites and metabisulphites are commonly used antioxidants in aqueous injections. Antioxidants must be carefully selected for use in injections to avoid interaction with the drug. Injections may, in addition to antioxidants, also contain chelating agents such as EDTA or citric acid, which remove trace elements.

Buffers

The ideal pH of parenteral products is pH 7.4. If the pH is above pH 9, tissue necrosis may result, while below pH 3, pain and phlebitis can occur.

Buffers are included in injections to maintain the pH of the packaged product. Changes in pH can arise through interaction between the product and the container. Acetate, citrate and phosphate buffers are commonly used in parenteral products.

Tonicity-adjusting agents

Isotonic solutions have the same osmotic pressure as blood plasma and do not damage the membrane of red blood cells. Hypotonic solutions have a lower osmotic pressure than blood plasma and cause blood cells to swell and burst because of fluids passing into the cells by osmosis. Hypertonic solutions have a higher osmotic pressure than plasma and as a result, the red blood cells lose fluids and shrink. Thus the BP states that aqueous solutions for large-volume infusion fluids, together with aqueous fluids for subcutaneous, intradermal and intramuscular administration, should be made isotonic. Intrathecal injections must also be isotonic to avoid serious changes in the osmotic pressure of the cerebrospinal fluid. Aqueous hypotonic solutions are made isotonic by adding either sodium chloride, glucose or, occasionally, mannitol. The latter two agents are incompatible with some drugs. If the solution is hypertonic, it is made isotonic by dilution.

Injection solutions are often made isotonic with 0.9% sodium chloride solution. The amount of solute, or the required dilution necessary to make a solution isotonic, can be determined from the freezing point depression. The freezing point depression of blood plasma and tears is $-0.52°C$. Thus solutions that freeze at $-0.52°C$ have the same osmotic pressure as body fluids. Hypotonic solutions have a smaller freezing point depression and require the addition of a solute to depress the freezing point to $-0.52°C$.

The amount of adjusting substance added to these solutions may be calculated from the equation:

$$W = (0.5 - a)/b$$

Example 12.1

A 100-mL volume of a 2% w/v solution of glucose for intravenous injection is to be made isotonic by the addition of sodium chloride.

A 1% w/v solution of glucose depresses the freezing point of water by 0.1°C and a 1% solution of sodium chloride depresses the freezing point of water by 0.576°C.

The depression of freezing point of the unadjusted solution of glucose (*a*) will therefore be:

$$(a) = 2 \times 0.1 = 0.2$$

A 1% w/v solution of sodium chloride depresses the freezing point of water by 0.576°C (*b*).

Substituting these values for *a* and *b* in the aforementioned equation:

$$W = (0.52\ 0.2)/0.576 = 0.32/0.576 = 0.555$$

The intravenous solution thus requires the addition of 0.555 g of sodium chloride per 100 mL volume to make it isotonic with blood plasma.

---

where W = percentage concentration of adjusting substance in the final solution, a = freezing point depression of the unadjusted hypotonic solution, b = freezing point depression of a 1% weight in volume (w/v) concentration of the adjusting substance.

An extensive list of freezing point depression values is detailed in the *Pharmaceutical Codex* (1994: 53–64) (Example 12.1).

Other methods that are used to estimate the amount of adjusting substances required to make a solution isotonic include:
- Sodium chloride equivalents
- Molar concentrations
- Serum osmolarity.

Details of these methods are given in the *Pharmaceutical Codex* (1994: 64–67).

Units of concentration

The concentration of the components in parenteral products may be expressed in various ways (see also Ch. 1):
- *Percentage weight/volume.* Examples include: magnesium sulphate injection 50%, sodium chloride intravenous infusion 0.9%
- *Weight per unit volume.* Examples include: atropine sulphate 600 μg/mL or ephedrine hydrochloride injection 30 mg/mL
- *Millimoles per unit volume.* Examples include: potassium chloride solution, strong (sterile) contains 2 mmol each of K^+ and Cl^- per mL; Calcium Chloride Injection BP contains 2.5 mmol of Ca^{2+} and 5 mmol of Cl^- in 5 mL.

Example 12.2

Sodium chloride has one sodium and one chloride ion. Thus 1 mole of sodium chloride provides 1 mole of both sodium and chloride ions. The weight of sodium chloride, which provides a 1 mmol quantity is 58.5 mg. This weight corresponds to its relative molecular mass and provides 1 mmol of both sodium and chloride ions.

Magnesium chloride has one magnesium and two chloride ions. The weight in milligrams that provides 1 mmol of magnesium and 2 mmol of chloride ions is 203 mg. This weight corresponds to the relative molecular mass of this salt. The quantity of salt in milligrams containing 1 mmol of a particular ion can be determined by dividing the relative molecular mass of the salt by the number of the particular ions that it contains. Weights of common salts that provide 1 mmol are given in the 12th edition of the *Pharmaceutical Codex* (1994: 49–50).

During the formulation of injections and infusions, the units of interest are the ions of electrolytes and the molecules of non-electrolytes. For molecules, 1 millimole (mmol) is the weight in milligrams corresponding to its relative molecular mass. A mole of an ion is its relative atomic mass weighed in grams. The number of moles of each of the ions of a salt in solution depends on the number of each ion in the molecule of the salt (Example 12.2).

Special injections

These are more complex formulations than solutions for injection.

Suspensions

Suspensions for injection contain <5% of drug solids with a mean particle diameter within the range 5–10 μm. Owing to the presence of particles in these formulations, these injections are more difficult to process and sterilize than solutions for injection. During the manufacture of suspensions for injection, the components are prepared and sterilized separately. They are then aseptically combined (see Ch. 19). The final product cannot be filter sterilized, owing to the presence of particles in the formulation. Powders for use in sterile suspensions can be sterilized by gas, but gas residues must be avoided.

Dried injections

With these products, the dry sterile powder is aseptically added to a sterile vial. Alternatively, a sterile filtered solution can be freeze dried in a vial. The dry drug powder is reconstituted with a sterile vehicle before use.

Non-aqueous injections

Drugs that are insoluble in an aqueous vehicle can be formulated in solution using an oil as the vehicle. Several oils are used in these formulations, including arachis oil and sesame oil, which are easily metabolized. These viscous injections give a depot effect with slow release of the drug, and are administered by intramuscular injection.

Large-volume parenteral products

These are formulated as single-dose injections that are administered by intravenous infusion. They are sterile aqueous solutions or emulsions, with Water for Injections as the main component. It is important that they are free of particles. During the administration of these fluids, additional drugs are often added to the fluids (see Ch. 11). This may be carried out by the injection of small-volume parenteral products to the administration set of the fluid, or by the 'piggyback' method. In this procedure, a second, but smaller, volume infusion of an additional drug is added to the intravenous delivery system.

Large-volume parenteral products include:
- Infusion fluids to deliver drugs or restore fluid or electrolyte imbalance
- Total parenteral nutrition (TPN) solutions
- Intravenous antibiotics
- Patient-controlled analgesia
- Dialysis fluids
- Irrigation solutions.

All of these products have direct contact with blood or are introduced into a body cavity.

Large-volume parenteral fluids must be terminally heat sterilized. While Water for Injections is the main component of these products, they also incorporate other ingredients including:
- Carbohydrates, e.g. dextrose, sucrose and dextran
- Amino acids
- Lipid emulsions which contain vegetable or semisynthetic oil
- Electrolytes such as sodium chloride
- Polyols, including glycerol, sorbitol and mannitol.

Most large-volume parenteral fluids are clear aqueous solutions, except for the oil-in-water emulsions. The production of emulsions for infusion is highly specialized as they are destabilized by heat.

Production of large-volume parenteral products

The fluids are produced and filled into containers in a high-standard clean room environment (see Ch. 17). The use of stringent quality assurance procedures is essential to ensure the quality of the products.

In commercial manufacturing facilities, the fluids are packaged from a bulk container into the product container using high-speed filling machines. Just before the fluid enters the container, particulate matter is removed from the fluid by passing it through an in-line membrane filter. Immediately after filling, the neck of each glass bottle is sealed with a tight-fitting rubber closure that is kept in place with a crimped aluminium cap. The outer cap is also aluminium, and an outer tamper-evident closure is used.

When using plastic bags, the preformed plastic bag is aseptically filled and immediately heat sealed. As an alternative, a blow-fill-seal system can be used. Blow-fill-seal production decreases the problems with product handling, cleaning and particulate contamination. Following filling of the product into containers, the fluids are examined for particulate matter and the integrity of container closures established.

Moist heat is used to sterilize parenteral products, irrigation solutions and dialysis fluids as soon as possible after the containers have been filled. Plastic containers must be sterilized with an over-pressure during the sterilization cycle to avoid the containers bursting.

Containers and closures

Large-volume parenteral fluids are packaged into:
- Glass bottles
- Polyvinyl chloride (PVC) collapsible bags
- Semi-rigid polythene containers.

The containers and closures that are used for packaging parenteral products must:
- Maintain the sterility of the packed fluids
- Withstand sterilization
- Be compatible with the packed fluid
- Allow withdrawal of the contents.

Glass bottles are rarely used these days, but may be used for products that are incompatible with plastic containers. If used, they require the use of an air inlet filter device for pressure equilibration within the container. Particles of glass can be released into the injection fluids. Damage to the neck of the bottles may result in contamination of the container contents from the external environment. Owing to these difficulties with glass containers, plastic containers have become widely used.

PVC collapsible bags are used to package most infusion fluids. They are designed with a port for the attachment of the administration set and an additive port for the addition of small-volume parenteral fluids.

PVC collapsible bags are:
- Resistant to impact
- Flexible and collapse during fluid administration and do not require an air inlet system.

The disadvantages of plastic bags are that:
- They permit a high moisture penetration
- They adsorb some drugs
- They require an extended sterilization time due to the heat resistance of the PVC
- Moist heat sterilization requires air ballasting to avoid pouch explosion.

Semi-rigid plastic containers are used for volumes of 100 mL for electrolyte solutions, 3 L for TPN solutions and up to 5 L for dialysis solutions.

Semi-rigid containers:
- Are more drug compatible than PVC containers
- Are difficult to break
- Do not fully collapse
- Need extended heat sterilization times
- Need air equilibration.

Semi-rigid bags are designed with two ports. One port allows the attachment of the administration set. The other port permits the addition of small-volume parenteral products or small-volume infusion fluids. They have a graduated scale that can be read either in an inverted or upright position (Fig. 12.3). To enable containers of large-volume parenteral fluids to be suspended from a drip stand for administration, bags are made with an eyelet opening that suspends the bag.

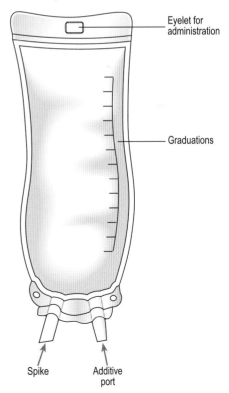

Eyelet for administration

Graduations

Spike

Additive port

Fig. 12.3 Semi-rigid infusion bag.

Administration of large-volume parenteral fluids

Most large-volume parenteral fluids are administered to the patient by a parenteral route using the standard infusion set specified in British Standard 2463 (Part 2, 1989). These sets are packaged as sterile units intended for single use (Fig. 12.4). Fluid moves through them by gravity.

Labelling

Batch-produced products have identical labels attached to both the product and the outer packaging carton that is used for transport. With flexible plastic containers, the labelling requirements are commonly printed directly on to the container before filling. With bags containing TPN fluids, a label is placed on the bag itself, and an identical label is attached to the outer plastic cover on the bag. Labels are attached to infusion fluid containers. The labels on parenteral fluids should include the following details:

- Product identity and details of the contained volume
- Solution strength in terms of the amount of active ingredient in a suitable dose-volume
- Batch number and product expiry date

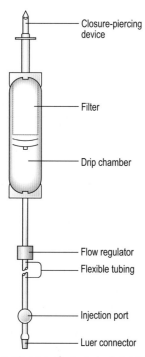

Fig. 12.4 Diagram of a typical administration set.

- Closure-piercing device
- Filter
- Drip chamber
- Flow regulator
- Flexible tubing
- Injection port
- Luer connector

- Storage requirements
- For TPN solutions, the name of the patient, the unit number, ward and infusion rate.

Containers often carry a warning label to discard the remaining product when treatment is completed.

Aseptic dispensing

Most parenteral fluids are terminally moist-heat sterilized. However, some products are aseptically compounded from sterile ingredients in the hospital pharmacy. These products are prepared and dispensed for individual patients. Examples of aseptically prepared products are TPN fluids (see Ch. 15), and the aseptic reconstitution of freeze-dried formulations. These freeze-dried products are often reconstituted using either water for injections, or 0.9% sodium chloride injection. Aseptic dispensing is performed in a Grade A clean room environment or a Grade A isolator chamber (see Ch. 11). The dispensing of these products relies on good aseptic procedures to ensure the sterility of the product. Owing to the absence of terminal sterilization, it is important that manufacture is performed using rigorous quality assurance procedures. Aseptically dispensed products are given a very limited expiry time.

Admixtures

These are prepared by adding at least one sterile injection to an intravenous infusion fluid for administration. The injections to be added are packed in an ampoule or vial, or may be reconstituted from a solid. These additions should be carried out using aseptic procedures in a Grade A environment within an isolator cabinet or clean room facility. This environment is required to maintain the sterility of the product, and avoid contamination of the product with particulate matter, microorganisms and pyrogens. Following the additions, a sealing cap may be placed over the additive port of the infusion bag to prevent further, potentially incompatible, additions at ward level. Hospital pharmacies often have a centralized intravenous additive service (CIVAS), as detailed in Chapter 17. These facilities ensure that additions to infusion fluids are carried out in a suitable environment.

Infusion devices

There are situations that require strict control of the volume of fluids that are infused into a patient. Accurate flow control with infusion devices is vital for patient safety and for optimum efficacy of the infusion. A range of delivery systems is available that regulates the volume of fluid administered, and are used both in the hospital and for the self-administration of fluids by patients at home.

The selection of an infusion device for the self-administration of medicines by patients requires careful consideration of several factors including:

- Delivery volume and control of flow rate
- Complexity of the administration procedure
- Type of therapy being administered
- Frequency of dosing
- Reservoir volume available in the infusion device.

Irrigation solutions

These solutions are applied topically to bathe open wounds and body cavities. They are sterile solutions for single use only. Examples of irrigation fluids are 0.9% w/v sodium chloride solution or sterile water for irrigation. Most irrigation fluids are now available in rigid plastic bottles. Urological irrigation solutions are used for surgical procedures. They are usually sterile water or sterile glycine solutions and are used to remove blood and maintain tissue integrity during an operation.

Water for irrigation is sterilized distilled water that is free of pyrogens. The water is packed in containers and is intended for use on one occasion only. The containers are sealed and sterilized by moist heat.

Peritoneal dialysis fluids

Peritoneal dialysis involves the administration of dialysis solutions directly into the peritoneum by way of an indwelling catheter. The fluid is then drained after a 'dwell-time' to remove toxic waste products from the body. Peritoneal dialysis solutions are sterile solutions manufactured to the same standards as parenteral fluids. The composition of peritoneal dialysis fluid simulates potassium-free extracellular fluid. These fluids are packaged in volumes of 3–5 L in plastic containers that are similar to the bags used for TPN (see Ch. 15).

Haemodialysis

In this dialysis procedure, blood is removed and returned to the patient by way of a catheter, or a double needle arrangement, using a fistula where an artery and vein are joined together. The dialysis procedure involves the use of an artificial disposable membrane within a 'dialyser' machine that acts as an artificial kidney. An electrolyte fluid, simulating body fluid, bathes one side of the membrane, with blood from the patient on the other side. There is no direct contact between the blood and the dialyser fluid. Thus fluids for haemodialysis are not required to be sterile or free of pyrogens or particulate matter.

Blood products

These products are not usually identified as sterile products although they are commonly packaged as sterile large-volume parenteral fluids. These biological products include albumin, human plasma and blood protein fractions. All these products must be treated to inactivate virus contamination before packaging. This is usually achieved by specialized heat treatment or filtration. These products are unstable to heat sterilization. Therefore they are filter sterilized and then aseptically filled into containers in large-scale production facilities. Most of these products are packed as liquids, although a few blood protein fractions such as factor VIII and factor IX are freeze dried. The collection, management and distribution of these products is carried out by the blood transfusion service.

Key points

- Convention uses the term 'parenteral' for dosage forms which are placed directly into the body
- The three main routes are IV, IM and SC
- Parenteral products are sterile forms used for injection, infusion or implantation
- Small volumes are packed in glass or plastic ampoules
- Multiple-dose injections must have an antimicrobial preservative
- Water for Injections must be used as the aqueous ingredient in all injections
- Water for irrigation is used in large volumes to irrigate body cavities and other areas
- Pyrogens cause fever and must be eliminated from water for injections and water for irrigations
- Additives to injections include antimicrobial preservatives, antioxidants, buffers, tonicity adjusters and co-solvents
- Injection solutions for SC, intradermal, IM, intrathecal and large-volume IV use should be made isotonic
- Large-volume parenteral products, include infusion fluids, TPN, dialysis fluids and irrigation solutions
- All large-volume parenteral products must be sterilized after filling into their final containers
- Large-volume parenteral products may be packaged in glass bottles, semi-rigid or collapsible plastic containers
- When aseptic dispensing is required, rigorous quality assurance is essential and a short expiry date is given to the product

Chapter 13

Ophthalmic products

R. Michael E. Richards

STUDY POINTS

- The formulation, preparation and uses of ophthalmic preparations
- The packaging and labelling requirements for ophthalmic preparations
- Advising patients on the use of eye medication and on any adverse effects
- The anatomy and physiology of the eye in relation to the administration of medication and the wearing of contact lenses
- The properties of contact lenses in relation to their physicochemical composition
- The wearing of, and caring for, contact lenses and the various products available to facilitate comfort, effectiveness, convenience and safety
- The role of antimicrobial preservatives in ophthalmic products
- Advising patients on the possible adverse effects of concurrent medication and the sensible use of cosmetics when wearing contact lenses

Introduction

The human eye is a remarkable organ and the ability to see is one of our most treasured possessions. Thus the highest standards are necessary in the compounding of ophthalmic preparations and the greatest care is required in their use. It is necessary that all ophthalmic preparations are sterile and essentially free from foreign particles.

These preparations may be categorized as follows:

- Eye drops including solutions, emulsions and suspensions of active medicaments for instillation into the conjunctival sac
- Eye lotions for irrigating and cleansing the eye surface, or for impregnating eye dressings
- Eye ointments, creams, and gels containing active ingredient(s) for application to the lid margins and/or conjunctival sac
- Contact lens solutions to facilitate the wearing and care of contact lenses
- Parenteral products for intracorneal, intravitreous or retrobulbar injection
- Ophthalmic inserts placed in the conjunctival sac and designed to release active ingredient over a prolonged period
- Powders for the preparation of eye drops and eye lotions. Medicaments contained in ophthalmic products include:
- Anaesthetics used topically in surgical procedures
- Anti-infectives such as antibacterials, antifungals and antivirals
- Anti-inflammatories such as corticosteroids and antihistamines
- Antiglaucoma agents to reduce intraocular pressure, such as beta-blockers
- Astringents such as zinc sulphate
- Diagnostic agents such as fluorescein, which highlight damage to the epithelial tissue
- Miotics such as pilocarpine, which constrict the pupil and contract the ciliary muscle, increasing drainage from the anterior chamber
- Mydriatics and cycloplegics such as atropine, which dilate the pupil and paralyse the ciliary muscle, and thus facilitate the examination of the interior of the eye.

Anatomy and physiology of the eye

Figure 13.1 gives an indication of the relevance of the external structures of the eye and the structure of the eyelids to the application of medication and the wearing of contact lenses.

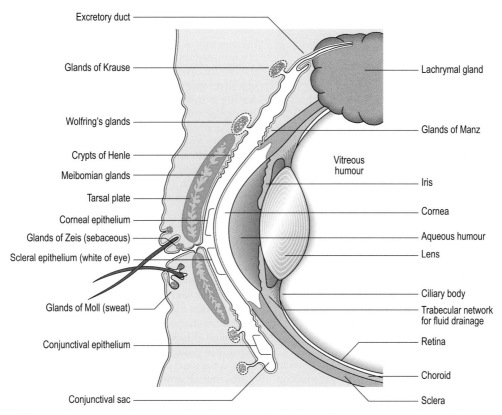

Fig. 13.1 Section of the eye showing the glands which produce the fluids that form the precorneal film and the tears, the epithelial sites of drug action and absorption and the internal sites of pharmacological action.

Formulation of eye drops

The components of an eye drop formulation are given here:
- Active ingredient(s) to produce desired therapeutic effect
- Vehicle, usually aqueous but occasionally may be oil
- Antimicrobial preservative to eliminate any microbial contamination during use and thus maintain sterility; it should not interact adversely with the active ingredient(s)
- Adjuvants to adjust tonicity, viscosity or pH in order to increase the 'comfort' in use and to increase the stability of the active ingredient(s); they should not interact adversely with other components of the formulation
- Suitable container for administration of eye drops which maintains the preparation in a stable form and protects from contamination during preparation, storage and use.

The single most important requirement of eye drops is that they are sterile. Historically, instances of microbially contaminated eye drops have been reported; the contaminating organism, *Pseudomonas aeruginosa*, is difficult to treat successfully and can cause loss of the eye.

Antimicrobial preservatives

Multiple-dose eye drops contain an effective antimicrobial preservative system, which is capable of withstanding the test for efficacy of antimicrobial preservatives of the *British Pharmacopoeia* (BP 2007). This ensures that the eye drops are kept sterile during use and will not introduce contamination into the eyes being treated. Normal healthy eyes are quite efficient at preventing penetration by microorganisms. Eyes that have damaged epithelia are compromised and may be colonized by microorganisms. This has to be guarded against. The lack of vascularity of the cornea and certain internal structures of the eye make it very susceptible and difficult to treat once infection has been established.

No single substance is entirely satisfactory for use as a preservative for ophthalmic solutions. The systems that

Labels in figure:
Excretory duct
Glands of Krause
Wolfring's glands
Crypts of Henle
Meibomian glands
Tarsal plate
Corneal epithelium
Glands of Zeis (sebaceous)
Scleral epithelium (white of eye)
Glands of Moll (sweat)
Conjunctival epithelium
Conjunctival sac
Lachrymal gland
Glands of Manz
Vitreous humour
Iris
Cornea
Aqueous humour
Lens
Ciliary body
Trabecular network for fluid drainage
Retina
Choroid
Sclera

Box 13.1 **Preservatives suitable for specific eye drops**

Benzalkonium chloride	Chlorhexidine acetate	Phenylmercuric nitrate[a]
0.01% w/v	0.01% w/v	0.002% w/v
Atropine sulphate	Cocaine	Tetracaine
Carbachol	Cocaine and homatropine	Chloramphenicol
Cyclopentolate		Fluorescein[b]
Homatropine		Hydrocortisone and neomycin
Hyoscine		Lachesine
Hypromellose		Neomycin
Phenylephrine		Sulfacetamide
Physostigmine		Zinc sulphate
Pilocarpine		Zinc sulphate and adrenaline
Prednisolone		

[a]The acetate may also be used.
[b]This is preferably used as single dose preparations.

have been used, based on work of the author and others in the 1960s, have formed the basis of effective preservation over the subsequent years.

Eye drops specifically formulated for use during intraocular surgery should not contain a preservative because of the risk of damage to the internal surfaces of the eye. Diagnostic dyes should preferably be supplied as single-dose preparations. Preservatives which are suitable for a selection of eye drops are given in Box 13.1.

Benzalkonium chloride

This quaternary ammonium compound is the preservative of choice. It is in over 70% of commercially produced eye drops and over a third of these also contain disodium edetate, usually at 0.1% w/v.

Benzalkonium chloride is not a pure material, but is a mixture of alkylbenzyldimethyl ammonium compounds. This permits a mixture of alkyl chain lengths containing even numbers of carbon atoms between 8 and 18 and results in products of different activities. The longer the carbon chain length, the greater the antibacterial activity but the less the solubility. Therefore the manufacturer should seek to maximize the activity within the constraints of solubility. This means maximizing the proportions of C_{12}, C_{14} and C_{16}. It should be noted that Benzalkonium Chloride BP contains 50% w/v benzalkonium chloride.

Benzalkonium chloride is well tolerated on the eye up to concentrations of 0.02% w/v but is usually used at 0.01% w/v. It is stable to sterilization by autoclaving. The compound has a rapid bactericidal action in clean conditions against a wide range of Gram-positive and Gram-negative organisms. It destroys the external structures of the cell (cell envelope). It is active in the controlled aqueous environment and pH values of ophthalmic solutions. Activity is reduced in the presence of multivalent cations (Mg^{2+}, Ca^{2+}). These compete with the antibacterial for negatively charged sites on the bacterial cell surface. It also has its activity reduced if heated with methylcellulose or formulated with anionic and certain concentrations of nonionic surfactants. Benzalkonium chloride is incompatible with fluorescein (large anion) and nitrates and is sorbed from solutions through contact with rubber.

The antibacterial activity of benzalkonium is enhanced by aromatic alcohols (benzyl alcohol, 2-phenylethanol and 3-phenylpropanol) and its activity against Gram-negative organisms is greatly enhanced by chelating agents such as disodium edetate. These agents chelate the divalent cations, principally Mg^{2+}, of Gram-negative cells. These ions form bridges and bind the polysaccharide chains, which protrude from the outer membrane of these cells. Thus the integrity of the membrane is compromised and the benzalkonium chloride activity enhanced. This is particularly valuable in preserving against contamination with *Pseudomonas aeruginosa*.

The surface activity of benzalkonium chloride may be used to enhance the transcorneal passage of non-lipid-soluble drugs such as carbachol. Care must be taken since the preservative can solubilize the outer oily protective layer of the precorneal film. This film has an internal mucin layer in contact with the corneal and scleral epithelia, a middle aqueous layer and an outer oily layer. The oil prevents excessive aqueous evaporation and protects the inner surface of the lids from constant contact with water. The blink reflex helps maintain the integrity of the precorneal film. For these reasons, it is important not to use benzalkonium chloride to preserve local anaesthetic eye drops which abolish the blink reflex. The combined effect of the two agents causes drying of the eye surface and irritation of the cornea.

Chlorhexidine acetate or gluconate

Chlorhexidine is a cationic biguanide bactericide with antibacterial properties in aqueous solution similar to benzalkonium chloride. Its activity is often reduced in the presence of other formulation ingredients. It is used at 0.01% w/v. Its antibacterial activity against Gram-negative bacteria is enhanced by aromatic alcohols and by disodium edetate. Activity is antagonized by multivalent cations. Stability is greatest at pH 5–6, but it is less stable to autoclaving than benzalkonium chloride. Chlorhexidine salts are generally well tolerated by the eye although allergic reactions may occur.

Chlorobutanol

This chlorinated alcohol is used at 0.5% w/v and is effective against bacteria and fungi. Chlorobutanol is compatible with most ophthalmic products. The main disadvantages are its volatility, absorption by plastic containers and lack of stability at autoclave temperatures.

Organic mercurials

Phenylmercuric acetate and nitrate and thiomersal are organic mercurials. They are slowly active, at concentrations of 0.001–0.004% w/v, over a wide pH range against bacteria and fungi. Absorption by rubber is marked.

The organic mercurials should not be used in eye drops which require prolonged usage because this can lead to intraocular deposition of mercury (mercurialentis). Allergy to thiomersal is also possible.

Tonicity

Where possible, eye drops are made isotonic with lachrymal fluid (approximately equivalent to 0.9% w/v sodium chloride solution). In practice, the eye will tolerate small volumes of eye drops having tonicities in the range equivalent to 0.7–1.5% w/v sodium chloride. Nevertheless, it is good practice to adjust the tonicity of hypotonic eye drops by the addition of sodium chloride to bring the solution to the tonicity of the lachrymal fluid. Some preparations are themselves hypertonic and so no adjustment should be made.

Viscosity enhancers

There is a general assumption that increasing the viscosity of an eye drop increases the residence time of the drop in the eye and results in increased penetration and therapeutic action of the drug. Most commercial preparations have their viscosities adjusted to be within the range 15–25 millipascal seconds (mPas). However, gently pressing downwards on the inside corner of the closed eye restricts the drainage channel into the nasal cavity and prolongs contact time. This has been recommended to increase the therapeutic index of antiglaucoma medications. Under normal conditions, a large proportion of a typical 50-µL drop will have drained from the conjunctival sac (capacity 25 µL) within 30 s. There will be no trace of the drop after 20 min.

Hypromellose

The hydroxypropyl derivative of methylcellulose is the most popular cellulose derivative employed for enhancing viscosity. It has good solubility characteristics (soluble in cold but insoluble in hot water) and good optical clarity. Typical concentrations in eye drop formulations are 0.5–2.0% w/v.

Polyvinyl alcohol

This is used at 1.4% w/v as a viscosity enhancer. It has a good contact time on the eye surface and good optical qualities. It withstands autoclaving and it can be filtered through a 0.22-µm filter.

Polyvinylpyrrolidone, polyethylene glycol and dextrin have also been used as viscolizing agents.

pH adjustment

The best compromise is required after considering the following factors:
- The pH offering best stability during preparation and storage
- The pH offering the best therapeutic activity
- The comfort of the patient.

Most active ingredients are salts of weak bases and are most stable at an acid pH but most active at a slightly alkaline pH.

The lachrymal fluid has a pH of 7.2–7.4 and also possesses considerable buffering capacity. Thus a 50-µL eye drop which is weakly buffered will be rapidly neutralized by lachrymal fluid. Where it is possible, very acidic solutions, such as adrenaline acid tartrate or pilocarpine hydrochloride, are buffered to reduce a stinging effect on instillation. Suitable buffers are shown in Box 13.2.

Antioxidants

Reducing agents are preferentially oxidized and are added to eye drops in order to protect the active ingredient from oxidation. Active ingredients requiring protection include

---

Box 13.2 Buffers suitable for some specific eye drops

Borate buffer (boric acid/borax): pH range 6.8–9.1
- Chloramphenicol eye drops: BP 1993 – pH 7.5
- Hypromellose eye drops: BPC 1973 – pH 8.4

Phosphate buffer (sodium acid phosphate/ sodium phosphate): pH range 4.5–8.5
- Neomycin eye drops: BPC 1973 – pH 6.5
- Prednisolone sodium phosphate eye drops: BPC 1973 – pH 6.6

Citrate buffer (citric acid/sodium citrate): pH range 2.5–6.5
- Benzylpenicillin eye drops – pH 6.0
- Idoxuridine eye drops – pH 6.0

adrenaline (epinephrine), proxymetacaine, sulfacetamide, tetracaine, phenylephrine, and physostigmine.

Sodium metabisulphite and sodium sulphite

Both may be used as antioxidants at 0.1% w/v. The former is preferred at acid pH and the latter at alkaline pH. Both are stable in solution when protected from light. Sodium metabisulphite possesses marked antimicrobial properties at acid pH and enhances the activity of phenylmercuric nitrate at acid pH. It is incompatible with prednisolone phosphate, adrenaline (epinephrine), chloramphenicol and phenylephrine.

Chelating agents

Traces of heavy metals can catalyse breakdown of the active ingredient by oxidation and other mechanisms. Therefore chelating agents such as disodium edetate may be included to chelate the metal ions and thus enhance stability. Disodium edetate is a very useful adjuvant to ophthalmic preparations at concentrations of up to 0.1% w/v to enhance antibacterial activity and chemical stability. It has also been used at higher concentrations as an eye drop for the treatment of lime burns in cattle.

Bioavailability

The effect of pH on the therapeutic activity of weak bases such as atropine sulphate has already been indicated under the section on pH adjustment. At acid pH, these bases exist in the ionized hydrophilic form. In order to penetrate the cornea, the bases need to be at alkaline pH so that they are in the unionized lipophilic form. Thus at tear pH (7.4) they are able to penetrate the outer lipid layer of the lipid–water–lipid sandwich, which constitutes the physicochemical structure of the cornea. Once inside the epithelium, the undissociated free base will partially dissociate. The water-soluble dissociated moiety will then traverse the middle aqueous stromal layer of the cornea. When the dissociated drug reaches the junction of the stroma and the endothelium it will again partially associate, forming the lipid-soluble moiety and thus cross the endothelium. Finally, the drug will dissociate into its water-soluble form and enter the aqueous humour. From here, it can diffuse to the iris and the ciliary body which are the sites of its pharmacological action (see Fig. 13.1). Thus the most effective penetration of the lipophilic–hydrophilic–lipophilic corneal membrane is by active ingredients having both hydrophilic and lipophilic forms. For example, highly water-soluble steroid phosphate esters have poor corneal penetration but the less water-soluble, more lipophilic steroid acetate has much better corneal penetration.

Storage conditions

To minimize degradation of eye drop ingredients, storage temperature and conditions must be considered at the time of formulation. The stability of several drugs used in eye drops is improved by refrigerated storage (2–8°C), e.g. chloramphenicol.

Containers for eye drops

Containers should protect the eye drops from microbial contamination, moisture and air. Container materials should not be shed or leached into solution, neither should any of the eye drop formulation be adsorbed or absorbed by the container. If the product is to be sterilized in the final container, all parts of the container must withstand the sterilization process.

Containers may be made of glass or plastic and may be single- or multiple-dose containers. The latter should not contain more than 10 mL. Both single-dose and multiple-dose packs must have tamper-evident closures and packaging.

Single-dose containers

The 'Minims' range is the most widely used type of single-dose eye drop container in the UK. It consists of an injection-moulded polypropylene container which is sealed at its base and has a nozzle sealed with a screw cap. This container is sterilized by autoclaving in an outer heat-sealed pouch with peel-off paper backing.

Plastic bottles

Most commercially prepared eye drops are supplied in plastic dropper bottles similar to the illustration in Figure 13.2. Bottles are made of polyethylene or polypropylene and are sterilized by ionizing radiation prior to filling under aseptic conditions with the previously sterilized preparation.

Glass bottles

Most extemporaneously prepared eye drops are supplied in 10-mL amber partially ribbed glass bottles.

The components of the eye dropper bottle are illustrated in Figure 13.3.

Bottles can be made of neutral glass and can be autoclaved more than once, or soda glass, which has had the internal surfaces treated during manufacture to reduce the release of alkali when in contact with aqueous solutions, but can only be autoclaved once. The teat can be made of good-quality natural or synthetic rubber. The former will withstand autoclaving at 115°C for 30 min but will not withstand the high temperatures of dry-heat sterilization.

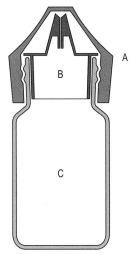

Fig. 13.2 Plastic eye drop bottle. (A) Rigid plastic cap. (B) Polythene friction plug containing baffle that produces uniform drops. (C) Polythene bottle.

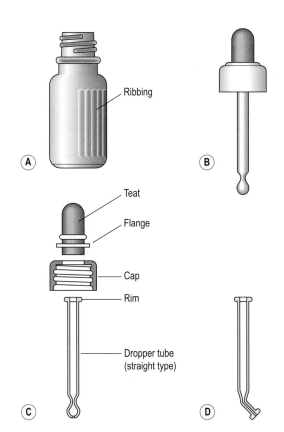

Fig. 13.3 Eye dropper bottle. (A) Bottle. (B) Assembled closure. (C) Components of closure. (D) Dropper tube (angled type).

The latter teats, made from silicone rubber, will withstand dry-heat sterilization and are suitable for use with oily eye drops. Silicone rubber is permeable to water vapour and for this reason aqueous eye drops in bottles having silicone rubber teats are given a limited shelf-life of 3 months. This can be lengthened by supplying the sterile eye drops in an eye drop bottle, sealed with an ordinary screw cap together with a separately wrapped and sterilized silicone rubber dropper unit. The dropper is carefully substituted for the cap when the eye drops are about to be used.

Teats and caps are used once only. All components are thoroughly washed with filtered distilled or deionized water, dried and stored in a clean area until required.

Rubber teats sorb preservatives and antioxidants during autoclaving and storage. It is necessary that individual studies are undertaken during formulation to help counteract preservative and antioxidant loss.

Preparation of eye drops

Extemporaneous preparation of eye drops involves the following:
- Preparation of the solution
- Clarification
- Filling and sterilization.

Preparation of the solution

The aqueous eye drop vehicle containing any necessary preservative, antioxidant, stabilizer, tonicity modifier, viscolizer or buffer should be prepared first. Then the active ingredient is added and the vehicle made up to volume.

Clarification

The BP has stringent requirements for the absence of particulate matter in eye drop solutions. Sintered glass filters or membrane filters of 0.45–1.2 µm pore sizes are suitable. The clarified solution is either filled directly into the final containers which are sealed prior to heat sterilization or temporarily filled into a suitable container prior to filtration sterilization. Clarified vehicle is used to prepare eye drop suspensions which are filled into final containers and sealed prior to sterilization.

Sterilization

This can take the form of:
- Autoclaving at 115°C for 30 min or 121°C for 15 min
- Filtration through a membrane filter having a 0.22 µm pore size into sterile containers using strict aseptic technique. Filling should take place under Grade A laminar airflow conditions (see Ch. 17)

95

Table 13.1 Labelling requirements for eye drop and eye ointment containers at the time of dispensing

Requirement	Include on label
State route of administration	'For use in the eye only'
Fully identify the product	The name and concentration of the active ingredient(s)
Statement on preservation	Confirm presence or absence of preservative
Directions for use	e.g. 'Add one drop to each eye morning and evening'
State an 'in use' expiry date	Day, month, year
Storage requirements	'Store in a cool place' or 'Protect from light'
Identify patient	Patient's name
Date of dispensing	Day, month, year

Note: When the stability of the final preparation requires it, eye drops may be provided in two containers as a dry powder and an aqueous vehicle. The labels should state 'Powder for eye drops' on one container and the directions for the preparation of the eye drops on the other package or container.
Based on the Department of Health guidance HSC(IS)122 1975, revised by the Royal Pharmaceutical Society of Great Britain 2001.

Box 13.3 Additional labelling requirements for use in specific locations

All locations

- Name and concentration of any antimicrobial present

Hospital: wards

- Patient's name. The eye to be treated. Date of opening bottle and/or date to discard (7 days later)

Hospital: operating theatres

- Single dose for once only use. Marked with indication of active ingredient and concentration. No preservative. Outer package fully labelled

Hospital: clinics

- Single dose or multidose used once only

Domiciliary

- 'Avoid contamination of contents during use'. 'Discard 28 days after opening'. 'Keep out of the reach of children'.

Note: If both eyes are to be treated and the patient has an open infection and/or medical opinion dictates, a separate bottle is supplied for each eye and labelled accordingly.

- Dry-heat sterilization at 160 °C for 2 h is employed for non-aqueous preparations such as liquid paraffin eye drops. Silicone rubber teats must be used.

Immediately following sterilization, the eye drop containers must be covered with a readily breakable seal, such as a viskring, to distinguish between opened and unopened containers.

Labelling of containers

Labelling requirements are summarized in Table 13.1 and Box 13.3.

Instillation of eye drops

Patients who have not used eye drops before need an explanation of how to instil the drops satisfactorily.
- Wash hands
- Tilt head back and with one hand gently pull down lower eyelid to form a pouch between the eye and the eyelid

- Hold dropper bottle (or separate eye dropper containing eye drops) above the eye, and drop a single drop into the preformed pouch. Do not touch the dropper on the eye or eyelid. (Using a well-illuminated mirror will help.) Administration aids are available to assist the self-administration of eye drops contained in plastic eye dropper bottles
- Release lower lid. Try not to blink more than usual as this removes the medicine from the eye
- Replace the dropper in the bottle or the cap on the bottle.

Formulation of eye lotions

The purpose of eye lotions is to assist in the cleaning of the external surfaces of the eye. This might be to help remove a non-impacted foreign body or to clean away conjunctival discharge. Eye lotions may also be used to impregnate eye dressings. Eye lotions intended for use in surgical or first-aid procedures should not contain antimicrobial preservatives and should be supplied in single-use containers. In keeping with their simple requirements, these preparations should have simple formulations and the most common eye lotion consists of sterile normal saline. This preparation typifies the requirements of an eye lotion which are:

- Sterile and usually containing no preservative
- Isotonic with lachrymal fluid
- Neutral pH
- Large volume but not greater than 200 mL
- Non-irritant to ocular tissue.

Labels

These should include:

- Title identifying the product and concentration of contents
- 'Sterile until opened'
- 'Not to be taken'
- 'Use once and discard the remaining solution'
- Expiry date.

Preserved eye lotion would need the additional labelling:

- 'Avoid contamination of contents during use'
- 'Discard remaining solutions not more than 4 weeks after first opening'.

The lotions should be supplied in coloured bottles and sealed to exclude microorganisms.

Powders for the preparation of eye drops and powders for the preparation of eye lotions

These powders are supplied in a dry, sterile form for dissolving or suspending in an appropriate vehicle at the time of use to provide a solution or suspension which complies with the requirements for eye drops or eye lotions as appropriate. The powders may contain suitable excipients to aid dissolution or dispersion, to adjust the tonicity and to improve stability. Unless an exception has been authorized, eye drops in the form of a suspension must pass the same particle size limit test as that applied to the size of particles in eye ointments (see later). In addition, single-dose powders for eye drops and eye lotions should either comply with the test for the uniformity of dosage of the *European Pharmacopoeia* (EP), or where appropriate, with the tests for uniformity of content and/or uniformity of mass.

Formulation of eye ointments

Eye ointments are popular and duplicate many of the therapeutic options offered by eye drops. Ointments have the disadvantage of temporarily interfering with vision, but have the advantage over liquids of providing greater total drug bioavailability. However, ointments take a longer time to reach peak absorption.

Eye ointments must be sterile and may contain suitable antimicrobial preservatives, antioxidants, and stabilizers. The *United States Pharmacopoeia* (USP 25) requires these ointments to contain one of the following antimicrobials: chlorobutanol, the parabens or the organic mercurials. In addition, such ointments should be free from particulate matter that could be harmful to the tissues of the eye. The EP and BP (2007) have limits for the particle size of incorporated solids. Each 10 µg of active solid should have no particles >90 µm, not more than 2 particles >50 µm and not more than 20 particles >25 µm.

The basic components of an eye ointment are:

Liquid paraffin	1 part
Wool fat	1 part (to facilitate incorporation of water)
Yellow soft paraffin	8 parts

Hard paraffin may be substituted as necessary to maintain an appropriate consistency in hot climates.

Containers for eye ointments

Eye ointments should be supplied in small sterilized collapsible tubes made of metal or a suitable plastic. The tube should not contain more than 10 g of preparation and must be fitted or provided with a nozzle of a suitable shape to facilitate application to the eye and surrounds without allowing contamination of the contents. The tubes must be suitably sealed to prevent microbial contamination.

Preparation of eye ointments

Eye ointments are normally prepared using aseptic techniques to incorporate the previously sterilized, finely powdered active ingredient or a sterilized concentrated solution of the medicament into the sterile eye ointment basis. Immediately after preparation, the eye ointment is filled into the sterile containers, which are then sealed so as to exclude microorganisms. The screw cap should be covered with a readily breakable seal.

All apparatus used in the preparation of eye ointments must be scrupulously clean and sterile. Certain commercial eye ointments may be sterilized in their final containers using ionizing radiation.

Preparation of eye ointment basis

The paraffins and the wool fat are heated together and filtered, while molten, through a coarse filter paper in a heated funnel into a container which can withstand dry-heat sterilization temperatures. The container is closed to exclude microorganisms. and together with contents, is maintained at 160°C for 2 h.

Ophthalmic inserts

These are sterile solid or semi-solid preparations for insertion in the conjunctival sac. They contain a reservoir of active material which is slowly released from a matrix or through a rate-controlling membrane over a known time period. Ophthalmic inserts each have their own sterile container which is labelled to state the total quantity of active substance per insert and, where applicable, its rate of release. The EP requires that, in the manufacturing of ophthalmic inserts, appropriate product dissolution behaviour is demonstrated.

Monitoring of eye preparations for adverse effects

Pharmacists should be available to counsel patients on the use of their eye medication and advise them about any adverse effects they may experience while using their medicines. Failing to use eye medication appropriately may also have serious consequences. It is important that the pharmacist is able to support the patient in using their medicine correctly. The pharmacist should also be alert to notice any signs/symptoms of adverse effects that the patient may be experiencing resulting from medication, in order to give appropriate and timely advice. Table 13.2 indicates the signs/symptoms of adverse effects, which may occur with eye preparations used in the treatment of primary open angle glaucoma. In addition to adverse effects associated

Table 13.2 Signs/symptoms of adverse effects which may occur with treatment for primary open angle glaucoma

Drugs used	General signs/symptoms of adverse effects	
Dose frequency as solutions/suspensions	Objective signs	Subjective signs
Beta-blockers	Blood pressure – hypotension	Difficulties in breathing, dry eyes
Timolol 2 × daily	Heart rate – slowed	Itchy and watery eyes
Timolol gel 1 × daily		Pain after instillation
Betaxolol 2 × daily		Blurring of vision
Carteolol 2 × daily		Palpitations
Levobunolol 1 or 2 × daily		Headaches, dizziness, anxiety
Metipranolol 2 × daily		
Parasympathomimetics (Miotics)	Heart rate – rarely affected	Variable blurring of vision
Pilocarpine 4 × daily		Reduction in night vision
Ocusert-Pilo[a] weekly		Transient headache
A slow-release gel formulation[a] 24-hourly		Ocular and periorbital pain
		Twitching eyelids
		Sweating, gastrointestinal upsets – rare
Sympathomimetics	Heart rate – quickened	Smarting and redness of eye
	Blood pressure – hypertension	Itchy, watery eyes
Adrenaline (epinephrine) 2 × daily	Conjunctival deposits of oxidized adrenaline[b]	Nasal obstruction
Guanethidine 2 × daily	Conjunctival fibrosis on prolonged guanethidine use[b]	Dilated pupil, could precipitate acute glaucoma – dangerous
Dipivefrine[a] 2 × daily		Headache, blurring vision

[a]These formulations can reduce adverse effects.
[b]These are specific effects.

with the eye, it should be noted that undesirable systemic effects can also occur with eye medication. Such systemic effects have been reported for certain potent ophthalmic medicines. This is due to excess solution draining from the eye surface through two small channels, the lachrymal canaliculi, into the lachrymal sac and on via the nasolachrymal duct and the gastrointestinal tract. Consequently, it is necessary to seek to avoid the instilling of excess eye drops.

Patients who are using an eye drop preparation for a chronic condition may become sensitive to the preservative in the formulation. This may also happen with contact lens products. Changing to a formulation having the same active ingredient but having a different or no preservative should solve the problem.

Contact lenses and their solutions

The ready accessibility of the eye and its external structures facilitates the fitting and wearing of lenses on the precorneal film and on the surface of the eye. Optometrists prescribe and fit contact lenses and monitor their use. Pharmacists should refer patients having persistent problems with wearing their lenses to their optometrist.

Popularity, problems, risks

The popularity of contact lenses results from their cosmetic appeal, optical advantages and their usefulness in sporting activities. Many prefer extended-wear soft lenses to daily-wear soft and hard lenses because of their relative convenience.

The problems that occur with the wearing of contact lenses result from inadequate education of the wearer about lens care. Extended-wear lenses in particular have been marketed in a manner which maximizes the volume of sales at the expense of adequate consumer education. That is, the marketing of lenses has overemphasized the convenient and carefree aspects of overnight lenses to the extent of trivializing the wearing of contact lenses. This has often resulted in poor patient compliance with suggested regimes of lens wear and care. It is estimated that more than 50% of those who wear contact lenses care for them unhygienically.

The risks associated with the wearing of contact lenses include recurrent corneal abrasions, corneal scarring and corneal vascularization. However, the most serious complication is microbial ulcerative keratitis or corneal ulcer, caused by microbial invasion of the cornea. Left untreated, this can lead to loss of vision. Fortunately, the natural defences of the cornea are very effective and the normal cornea resists microbial infection as long as the surface epithelium is intact.

It has been shown that the risk of corneal ulcers is 9–15 times greater for extended-wear lenses worn overnight than for daily-wear soft lenses worn only during the day. The risk increases with the number of consecutive days that lenses are worn without removal.

A serious, but fairly rare, complication that can arise from using non-sterile water in the care of lenses is infection with the free-living opportunistic pathogen *Acanthamoeba*. This is found in most soil and water habitats. *Acanthamoeba* keratitis is hard to diagnose and to treat and can lead to serious loss of vision. *Acanthamoeba* infection has also resulted from wearing soft lenses while bathing in a Jacuzzi; consequently, this practice is contraindicated.

The aim of formulators and providers of contact lens systems must be to supply the safest possible system with known and acceptable risks; that is, both convenience and safety must be the aim.

Relevant properties of the eye
Anatomy and physiology

Figure 13.1 indicates the structures of the eye which are particularly relevant to the use of topical medications, contact lenses and contact lens products. First, it is important to note that the cornea, the lens and the humour compartments are avascular, and that this property facilitates the transmission of light and vision. Second, exchange of nutrients and waste products in these situations takes place almost entirely by diffusion processes, through the aqueous humour, through the lens and cornea and through the lachrymal fluid. Contact lenses reduce the diffusion of oxygen to the cornea, and thus can affect corneal metabolism.

Secretions

The secretions of the eye have an important role and influence on the wearing of contact lenses. Lachrymal fluid, commonly known as *tears*, performs the important functions of lubricating, hydrating, cleaning and disinfecting the anterior surface of the eye. The latter function is performed by the enzyme lysozyme (1,4-*N*-acetylglycosaminidase) which catalyses the hydrolysis of 1,4-glycosidic linkages between *N*-acetyl muramic acid and *N*-acetyl-glucosamine in the peptidoglycan layer of the bacterial cell wall. The peptidoglycan layer of Gram-positive cells is accessible to the action of lysozyme.

The fluid forming the precorneal film is produced by differing groups of glands. It contains mucus (Henle and Manz), water (Krause and Wolfring) and oil (Meibomian, Moll and Zeis). These fluids are stratified in three distinct layers. The surface-active mucoid layer spreads on the corneal surface and associates with the intermediate aqueous layer externally. The aqueous layer is surfaced with an oily layer which lubricates and protects the mucous membranes of the internal lid surfaces.

Tear electrolyte content

This is broadly similar to that of serum, except that the potassium ion is approximately four to six times greater (24 mEq/L compared with 4–6 mEq/L in serum). The protein content of tears is mainly albumin and globulin and is approximately a 10th of that in serum (0.7% compared with 7%).

Tear production

Tears are produced by the lachrymal glands in response to four distinct types of stimuli: emotional via psychological factors, sensory via external irritants, continuous via automatic nervous control and systemic via chemicals in the bloodstream affecting the nerves innervating the lachrymal glands.

Tear pH

This is slightly alkaline at 7.2. Tears have sufficient buffering capacity to adjust rapidly the pH of small volumes of weakly buffered solutions to pH 7.2.

Eyelids

These perform a protecting and a cleaning function. The outer margins of the eyelids close slightly before the inner margins and sweep the fluids across the eye towards the lachrymal canaliculi at the inner angle of the eye from where it can pass via the lachrymal sac into the nasal cavity and gastrointestinal tract. Systemic absorption of excess eye medicament may take place through this mechanism.

Bacterial flora

There is a common misconception that lachrymal fluid is sterile. It has been known since 1908 that staphylococci and diphtheroids can be found regularly in normal conjunctiva. Gram-negative enteric bacilli have also been isolated from the conjunctivas and lids of about 5% of people. This shows that care is necessary when wearing contact lenses to avoid abrading the corneal epithelium.

Contact lenses

Sir John Herschel used a refractive glass shell in 1823 to protect the cornea from a diseased lid. Dr Eugen Fickfirst used the term 'contact lens' in 1887. Fick's blown glass lenses were intended to correct defective vision. In 1948 Tuohy introduced the hydrophobic hard plastic corneal lens, and in 1962 soft pliable lenses were introduced as the result of work in Prague University. These lenses have been very popular. Gas-permeable hard lenses have also been introduced which allow oxygen perfusion to the cornea. These lenses are more comfortable than the original hard lenses. The first extended-wear lenses were introduced in 1981.

The aim in making contact lenses is to produce lenses which will:

- Correct the patient's vision
- Maintain their position on the eye
- Allow respiration of the cornea
- Permit free flow of tears round or through the lens
- Not release toxic substances
- Not introduce microbial contamination
- Be wearable throughout the day
- Be easy to handle and economical to use.

Hard lenses

Polymethylmethacrylate (PMMA) or 'Perspex' has optical properties similar to spectacle crown glass. PMMA has hydrophobic properties conferred by the large proportion of methyl groups compared with hydrophilic carboxy ester groups. This means that lachrymal fluid does not readily wet lenses made of this material. Therefore the lenses need to be wetted before mounting on the precorneal film to reduce or eliminate patient discomfort. Hence the need for a wetting solution to facilitate wear, and the need for a storage, hydrating, decontaminating solution to facilitate care of the lenses when not being worn. The original hard lens composition had some major disadvantages for the wearer. Free passage of oxygen and carbon dioxide to and from the corneal epithelium could not take place. Corneal oedema and distortion were a common result. Thus modern lenses have been designed to be gas permeable. These lenses are physiologically more user-friendly and have greater wearer acceptance.

The original gas-permeable lenses consisted of cellulose acetate butyrate (CAB), which was readily wettable and proved quite acceptable. More recently, lenses based on silicone and fluorine have been produced which have greater gas permeability. Silicone methacrylate copolymers are very popular. The silicone composition controls the permeability properties and the PMMA composition controls the degree of rigidity. Similarly, fluorosilicone methacrylate copolymers, which have very high oxygen permeability properties and good wetting properties, are proving to be popular. These gas-permeable lenses are cared for using hard lens solutions. These lenses are less subject to deposits of lipids, protein and other substances from the lachrymal fluid than soft lenses. They also have better optical qualities and are generally easier to care for.

Soft lenses

Soft lenses are made from the hydroxyethyl ester of polymethacrylic acid (poly-HEMA). The large number of polar hydroxyl groups confers hydrophilic properties to the polymer. Poly-HEMA is flexible and can absorb about 47% of its own weight of water. Thus lenses of this material are comfortable and easy to wear but more difficult to care for than hard lenses. A particular problem is uptake of antibacterial preservatives and subsequent release and irritancy during wear. Although a wetting solution is not needed, cleaning, storing, hydrating and decontaminating functions are required of solutions.

Copolymers of poly-HEMA with vinylpyrrolidine (VP) are also produced, which can absorb up to 80% by weight of water, depending on the HEMA/VP ratio. The higher water content lenses have the advantage of greater gas permeability and comfort than the poly-HEMA lenses which may occasionally cause corneal oedema. However, they are more fragile and difficult to care for than poly-HEMA, have a greater tendency to attract deposits, more solution problems and less precise optical properties.

Disposable lenses

Disposable lenses may be discarded after 1 month, 1 week or even 1 day. The latter would obviate the need for the use of solutions, and theoretically increase the safety and acceptability of lens wear. However, the original intention of these lenses was for extended wear, without removal. It has already been pointed out that the additional risks that are associated with extended wear makes this an unattractive and even a dangerous practice. These lenses would seem to offer the greatest advantage to those people who wear lenses on an irregular basis for social and sporting activities, and for those children who may need soft lenses.

Hard lens solutions

A 'wetting solution' and a 'soaking/storing/decontaminating solution' are required for the wear and routine care of hard lenses. The first is suitable for placing in the eye, but the second must not have contact with the eye.

Wetting solution
Purpose

- Achieves rapid wetting by the lachrymal fluid and thus promotes comfort
- Facilitates insertion of lens
- Provides cushioning and lubrication
- Enables cleaning after removal
- Must be non-irritant during daily use.

Formulation

- Wetting and viscolizing agents – polyvinyl alcohol and hypromellose
- Viscosity 15–20 mPas for comfort
- pH 6.8
- Tonicity 0.9–1.1% sodium chloride
- Antimicrobials – benzalkonium chloride 0.004% plus disodium edetate 0.1%.

Storing solutions
Purpose

- Achieves cleaning and microbial inactivation
- Hydrating.

Formulation

- Surface-active agent not inactivating antimicrobials
- pH 7.4
- Antimicrobials – benzalkonium chloride 0.01% plus disodium edetate 0.1%.

Soft lens solutions

Cleaning solutions
Purpose

- To remove deposits such as lipoprotein adhering to the lens after wear.

Formulation

- Viscolizing surface-active agent such as hypromellose to enable suitable gentle friction with fingertips
- Antibacterial – fast-acting benzalkonium chloride 0.004% may be used if contact time is only 20–30 s.

Storing solutions
Purpose

- Hydrating
- Cleaning
- Inactivation of microbial contamination.

Formulation

- Isotonic ≡ 0.9% w/v sodium chloride
- Antibacterial.

Hydrogen peroxide – was introduced into commercially available care systems in 1984. Hydrogen peroxide is a powerful oxidizer and this is the source of its antimicrobial activity. It has good activity against *Acanthamoeba*.

$$2H_2O_2 > 2H_2O + O_2 + Energy$$

Decomposition is more rapid at alkaline than acid pH and many substances catalyse the reaction. These properties are utilized in the formulation of storage, disinfecting and cleaning solutions. For example, a solution containing 3% hydrogen peroxide at acid pH is used to disinfect lenses over a period of 6 h. This is then followed by suitable inactivation with sodium pyruvate, platinum or the enzyme catalase, to facilitate subsequent safe wearing of the lenses. The procedure is referred to as the *two-step system* because a separate neutralization step follows the disinfecting step. One-step systems have also been developed for greater patient convenience. The inactivating substance is incorporated with the 3% hydrogen peroxide and the lenses in the disinfecting solution. This system needs to be calibrated to slowly neutralize hydrogen peroxide, but to allow it to have antimicrobial activity over a 6 h period to ensure effectiveness against *Acanthamoeba* cysts. Some commercial systems may neutralize the effect of the hydrogen peroxide over a period of 30 min or so, which is too rapid to guarantee effectiveness.

Polyquad – a polyquaternium compound is used as an antimicrobial in soft lens solutions because it is not sorbed by lenses and it has low toxicity to corneal and ocular tissues.

(Thermal disinfection is an alternative disinfection process and the American FDA stipulates heating the lenses in a suitable solution in a lens case at a minimum of 80°C for 10 min. Heating reduces the life of the lens and it is also inconvenient.)

Enzyme protein digest

Purpose

- Occasional cleaning procedure followed by suitable washing and cleansing before wear. Frequency will vary with the individual and his/her state of health. Influenza or hay fever, for example, will increase the need.

Formulation

- Proteolytic enzyme, such as papain, as a solution tablet to produce a suitable solution when dissolved in a stated volume of sterile aqueous vehicle.

Lipid digest or combined protein and lipid digest systems are also available.

All-purpose solutions

The all-purpose solutions initially represented a compromise for hard lens wearers finding it difficult to comply with a two-solution regimen. Single-solution lens care systems are now widely available for use with soft lenses, which incorporate an enzyme cleaner combined with a disinfection solution. For example, the serine protease subtilisin A, obtained from the bacterium *Bacillus subtilis*, is used in the presence of hydrogen peroxide to remove protein contamination from contact lenses. Certain all-purpose lens solutions incorporate polyhexamide (polyhexamethylene biguanide) 0.00006–0.0004% as the antimicrobial agent. It is reported to be active against a wide range of bacteria and against *Acanthamoeba*.

All-purpose solutions for soft lenses have become very popular.

Containers

Contact lens solutions are usually packed in plastic containers. It is imperative that the low concentrations of antimicrobials present in these products are not reduced to ineffective levels due to sorption effects with the plastic.

Contact lens storage cases are also of importance to the contact lens wearer. It is important that these containers are kept in a hygienic condition by keeping them scrupulously clean and using the disinfecting/storage solutions strictly in accordance with the manufacturers' instructions. Storage cases should be changed periodically.

Advice to patients

General considerations

Contact lens wearers presenting at the pharmacy with a persistent red eye indicating an infection should not be recommended antibacterial eye drops. They should be referred to an ophthalmologist. This is to guard against the possibility that the person has an infection with *Acanthamoeba*. Such an infection would be more difficult to diagnose after partial treatment.

Disease states leading to a dry eye syndrome such as Sjögren syndrome, which is mostly confined to menopausal women who have osteoarthritis, will also adversely affect the ability of a person to wear contact lenses.

Hard lenses, and to a lesser extent soft lenses, interrupt the oxygen supply to the cornea and with prolonged wear produce increasing hypoxia. After approximately 16 h of wear, this corneal hypoxia results in a dip in the corneal glycogen level with resultant oedema. Irritation, itchiness, photophobia, and blurred vision can result. The patient should be advised not to over-wear the lenses and they may also be recommended to instil sterile sodium chloride 2% w/v every 3–4 h, after the lenses have been removed, until the oedema has resolved. They should be warned that the hypertonic drops may cause temporary stinging on instillation.

Adverse effects of medicines

Pharmacists should be aware that many medicines taken systemically can also cause problems for wearers of contact lenses and be prepared to offer appropriate counselling.

Certain medicines can affect the eye surface and lachrymal fluid production and thereby influence the comfort of contact lens wear. Medication having anticholinergic properties, such as sedative antihistamines, chlorphenamine, antispasmodics, hyoscine, tricyclic antidepressants and neuroleptics, can all reduce lachrymal fluid production. Diuretics will also reduce tear volume and topical timolol can cause transitory dry eyes. The consequent lack of lubrication may cause lens discomfort and increased lens deposits.

Oral contraceptives may cause corneal oedema, decreased aqueous and increased mucus and protein production, and thus lead to lens intolerance. Pregnancy may also be associated with increased lens awareness and discomfort, possibly associated with reduced tear flow and changes in corneal thickness and the curvature of the eye. Clomifene and primidone have also been reported to cause lid and corneal oedema.

Cholinergic drugs and also ephedrine and reserpine will increase tear volume. Aspirin produces low concentrations of salicylic acid in the lachrymal fluid. This can be absorbed by soft lenses and subsequently cause irritation. Isotretinoin may cause conjunctival inflammation and consequently cause discomfort to contact lens wearers.

Discolouration, via the lachrymal fluid, particularly with soft lenses, may occur with the administration of certain medicines such as labetalol, nitrofurantoin, phenothiazines, phenolphthalein, rifampicin, sulfasalazine and tetracyclines. Rifampicin for example will stain the lenses and tears orange.

Lenses must be removed before diagnostic dyes such as fluorescein are instilled. In fact, it is a general rule that patients should be counselled not to place any ophthalmic preparation on to the eyelids or surface of the eye, while contact lenses are in place. Certain eye drops may be instilled while hard lenses are being worn. Sterile 'Comfort drops' may be instilled while lenses are being worn to help maintain the hydration and lubrication of the eye surfaces and lenses when required. Numerous commercial solutions are available. The basic requirements are that the drops should be isotonic, have good wetting properties and be slightly viscous.

Concurrent use of cosmetics

Soft lenses should always be inserted before applying eye makeup but rigid gas-permeable lenses may be put on afterwards. All lenses should be put on before applying nail polish, hand creams, perfumes or using nail polish remover. Aerosol products should be used with caution so that spray does not get between the lens and the eye. All eye make-up should be water based and powders should be avoided. Mascara (not waterproof) should only be applied to the tips of the eyelashes.

The pharmacist should be aware of the various situations mentioned earlier when offering advice and discussing customers'/patients' questions.

Key points

- Ophthalmic preparations must be sterile
- Eye drops may be solutions, suspensions or emulsions and contain:
  - Active ingredient
  - Liquid vehicle free from particulate matter; particle size limits for suspensions
  - Antimicrobial preservative
  - Adjuvants: tonicity, viscosity, buffering, antioxidants, chelating, dispersing, emulsifying
- Eye drops are contained in a glass or plastic bottle
- Eye lotions are:
  - Isotonic
  - Neutral pH
  - Large volume but not greater than 200 mL
  - Non-irritant
  - Contained in a fluted, coloured bottle
- Eye ointments contain:
  - Semi-solid base
  - Active ingredient
  - Antimicrobial preservative
  - Adjuvants: antioxidants, stabilizers
- Eye ointments are:
  - Free from harmful particulate matter; particle size limits
  - Contained in a metal or plastic tube
- Ophthalmic inserts:
  - Contain a reservoir of active material
  - Incorporate a slow-release mechanism
- Properties of the eye affecting formulation of products include:
  - Anatomy and physiology
  - Secretions
  - Lids
  - Bacterial flora
- Contact lenses may be:
  - Hard lenses including gas permeable
  - Soft lenses including disposable
- Contact lens solutions may be:
  - Hard lenses – (i) wetting and cleaning; (ii) storing and disinfecting or (iii) all purpose
  - Soft lenses – (i) cleaning; (ii) storing and disinfecting or (iii) all purpose

- Enzyme cleaning agents are required for all lenses
- Pharmacists should be able to counsel patients on:
  - Possible adverse effects of eye medication
  - Common problems encountered by lens wearers
- Adverse effects of concurrent medications
- Concurrent use of cosmetics

Inhaled route

Peter M. Richards

The role of the pharmacist

Inhaled products are specialized dosage forms, which are designed to deliver medicines directly to the lung. A variety of inhaler devices are in use, all of which require the user of the inhaler to adopt an appropriate inhaler technique. Failure to use the correct inhaler technique will result in treatment failure. The pharmacist, who is usually the person who gives (dispenses) the inhaler to the patient, is ideally placed to demonstrate the appropriate inhalation technique for that inhaler. Using an inhaler is a skill, subject to the development of 'bad habits', which can lead to poor technique. Inhaler technique should therefore be regularly checked to ensure that the technique is optimal; again, the pharmacist is ideally placed to perform this function.

Pharmacists can also provide education to patients beyond a discussion of a patient's inhalers and other medicines, to include education about the patient's disease (e.g. asthma), and its management. Pharmacists also run asthma clinics and may do so as supplementary or independent prescribers. A few pharmacists have specialist respiratory consultant posts in secondary care. A pharmacist wishing to undertake a specialist role in respiratory medicine will need to gain appropriate experience, and undertake further training.

This chapter describes the most frequently prescribed inhaled therapies in the context of asthma and chronic obstructive pulmonary disease (COPD). The most widely prescribed inhaler devices are outlined along with instructions in their use.

Introduction

Many patients on inhaled therapy will be using more than one inhaler and may also have been prescribed a peak flow meter (PFM) to aid in monitoring their condition. In order for pharmacists to be able to provide useful education and advice to these patients, pharmacists will need to understand the condition being treated, and the role of the medicines and devices prescribed. This chapter will provide that understanding, in the context of the two most common airway diseases treated with inhaled medicines, namely asthma and COPD. It is beyond the scope of the chapter to discuss the diseases themselves, or the role of oral therapy and non-drug management of these conditions. It should be remembered that the most important interventions in COPD are smoking cessation and pulmonary rehabilitation.

There are significant differences in the way that inhalers are prescribed for asthma and COPD. In COPD, the emphasis of treatment is on the use of bronchodilators, and it may be appropriate for a COPD patient to have a long-acting inhaled beta-agonist without an inhaled steroid. This is different from asthma treatment where a long-acting beta-agonist should always be prescribed with an inhaled steroid. The scope of this chapter is limited to commonly used inhaled treatments and devices used for these inhaled treatments. By being familiar with national treatment guidelines for asthma and COPD, pharmacists can be assured that the advice that they give patients is likely to be consistent with that given by other healthcare professionals. These guidelines are BTS/SIGN Asthma Guidelines, which, at the time of writing are currently out for consultation and are due to be published in 2019 and NICE NG115 Chronic Obstructive Pulmonary disease: https://www.nice.org.uk/guidance/NG115.

Asthma is a very common condition in the UK, affecting at least 5% of adults and up to 10% of children; therefore many people will experience symptoms attributable to asthma at some time in their life.

COPD has been an under-publicized condition. Prevalence of COPD in the UK is thought to be 2–4% of the total population, with 1.5% of the population with diagnosed COPD. The decline in lung function leading to COPD is age-related but this decline can be rapidly accelerated in some smokers. COPD is thus an increasing problem in an ageing population.

Asthma and COPD are not mutually exclusive and some patients will have features of both diseases; this is often referred to as 'mixed disease'. The prevalence of asthma, COPD and related conditions means that pharmacists will not only frequently encounter patients on inhaled therapy during dispensing, but will also encounter patients on inhaled therapy when giving advice on the sale of over-the-counter medicines.

The inhaled route

The inhaled route delivers medicines to the lungs. Inhaled medicines may have a local effect on the lungs or may be absorbed to give a systemic effect. The inhaled route is generally used when the lung is the target organ, e.g.:

- The antibiotic colistimethate sodium is nebulized to treat lung infections associated with cystic fibrosis
- The antiviral zanamivir is presented as a dry-powder inhaler for treating influenza.

Using the inhaled route when the lung is the target organ has a number of advantages:

- A smaller dose can be used. The normal adult oral dose of salbutamol is 4 mg, but the normal inhaled dose of salbutamol is 200 µg
- The risk of unwanted systemic effects is reduced
- A faster onset of action may be achieved with some drugs, e.g. salbutamol
- Topically active drugs with poor oral bioavailability can be used.

The main disadvantage of the inhaled route is that inhaling a drug is more difficult than swallowing a tablet. Some drugs are ineffective by the inhaled route, e.g. theophylline.

Using the inhaled route does not result in the entire quantity of drug in the inhaler device reaching the lung. Even if an inhaler device is used perfectly, it is unlikely that any more than 20% of the drug reaches the lung. The majority of the rest of the drug remains in the oropharynx and is normally swallowed.

The lungs are designed to prevent the inhalation of anything other than gas. However, particles with a diameter of approximately 5 µm can be inhaled and have sufficient mass to settle in the lung. Particles larger than 10 µm remain in the oropharynx. Particles smaller than 1 µm are inhaled, but are then exhaled. Decreasing particle size increases the chance of penetration further down the tracheobronchial tree. It may be that a particle needs to be less than 3 µm to reach the 8th to 23rd branch generation. These particle sizes apply to the adult lung, and a smaller particle size of the order of 2.5 µm may be optimal in infant lungs.

The specific target in the lung for medicines used in asthma and COPD is the bronchiole. Branching from bronchi, bronchioles are the first airways in the lung not to contain cartilage and are less than 1 mm in diameter. The absence of cartilage means that smooth muscle contraction reduces the size of the airway. Inflammation also results in reduction in size of the airway (Fig. 14.1).

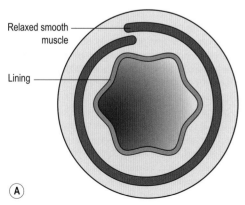

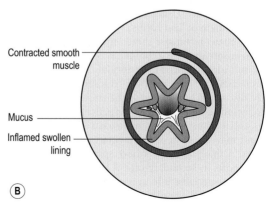

Fig. 14.1 Airways obstruction in asthma. (A) Unobstructed airway. (B) Obstructed airway.

Inhaled medicines used for asthma and COPD

Short-acting beta₂ agonists (SABAs)

Salbutamol and terbutaline are widely used SABAs. They act on beta₂ receptors in the smooth muscle of bronchioles to reverse bronchospasm. Symptoms caused by bronchospasm include wheeze, coughing, breathlessness, and a feeling of tightness of the chest. For this reason, SABAs are often referred to as 'relievers' and should be used 'as required' to relieve symptoms. If a reliever inhaler is required for asthma more than twice a week most weeks, the addition of a 'preventer' (usually a steroid) inhaler should be considered.

Points to note

- The inhaler itself is not dangerous – but asthma is potentially life-threatening
- Appropriate 'as required' use of a reliever inhaler provides a useful marker of the severity of the condition
- Frequent usage of a reliever inhaler may indicate severe uncontrolled asthma
- There is no risk that using the reliever inhaler whenever needed will result in a diminishing response, but worsening asthma will not respond to a reliever inhaler alone – additional treatment is required
- If the reliever inhaler is not relieving symptoms, urgent medical attention is required
- If reliever inhaler usage has increased, or is being used more than twice a week most weeks, review of treatment is required
- The reliever inhaler can be used immediately before sport/exercise to prevent exercise-induced asthma in susceptible individuals
- A reliever inhaler is normally blue.

Unwanted effects of inhaled beta₂ agonists are rare but tremor can occur.

SABAs are also prescribed for symptom relief in COPD.

Short-acting muscarinic antagonists (SAMAs)

The most commonly prescribed SAMA is ipratropium. Smooth muscle relaxation is achieved by opposing the parasympathetic nervous system. Ipratropium's role in COPD is now limited to being an alternative to salbutamol for as required relief of symptoms.

Long-acting beta₂ agonists (LABAs)

Salmeterol, formoterol and indacaterol are inhaled LABAs. Salmeterol and formoterol are licensed for use in both asthma and COPD and are used twice daily. Indacaterol is licensed for COPD only and is used once daily. These inhalers are sometimes referred to as 'protectors'.

Points to note

- LABAs should be used regularly and not on an 'as required' basis
- A reliever inhaler (SABA in asthma) should be used to relieve breakthrough symptoms
- For asthma, inhaled steroids (preventer inhalers) should be continued
- For COPD, it is appropriate to use a LABA without concomitant inhaled steroids

For COPD, a long-acting bronchodilator is the next step to a short-acting bronchodilator. A SABA (or SAMA) will also be required to relieve breakthrough symptoms.

Long-acting muscarinic antagonists (LAMAs)

Tiotropium bromide, glycopyrronium bromide and aclidinium bromide are inhaled LAMAs indicated for maintenance bronchodilator therapy in COPD. They are not licensed for asthma.

Inhaled corticosteroids (ICS)

The anti-inflammatory actions of steroids are able to control the inflammatory processes in asthma. No steroid inhaler is licensed for use in COPD. Two combination inhalers (LABA+ICS) at specific doses are licensed for COPD.

The inhaled route allows small doses of steroid to be used, minimizing the risk of systemic effects. The ideal inhaled steroid's properties would include:

- Poor absorption from the gastrointestinal tract to minimize systemic effects due to the swallowed portion
- Complete metabolism in the 'first pass' through the liver
- High topical activity
- Metabolism in the lung to inactive metabolites (absorption from the lung circumvents the 'first pass' through the liver).

Using a spacer device with the steroid inhaler, and/or rinsing the mouth with water and spitting immediately after using the inhaled steroid may reduce systemic effects and unwanted local effects in the mouth and throat.

Beclometasone, budesonide, fluticasone ciclesonide and mometasone are examples of inhaled steroids. They are used once or twice daily depending on their license. Inhaled steroids are often referred to as 'preventers'.

Inhaled steroids should normally be introduced:

- After a severe exacerbation of asthma
- If an asthmatic is using his short-acting beta$_2$ agonist more than twice a week
- If asthma is causing waking one night a week or more.

The aforementioned measures form the basis for assessing control of asthma; in addition, limitation of exercise due to asthmatic symptoms and measures of lung function can be considered.

Points to note

- Inhaled steroids should be used regularly, not on an 'as required' basis
- Inhaled steroids have no immediate effect
- Improved asthma control will take a minimum of 1–3 days, and it may be 14–28 days before maximum improvement is seen after starting or increasing the dose of inhaled steroid
- Beclometasone should be prescribed by brand name due to differences in bioavailability between brands
- Steroid inhalers are normally brown, orange or maroon.

Unwanted systemic effects of inhaled steroids are extremely rare provided that the total daily dose is less than the equivalent of 800–1000 µg beclometasone dipropionate.

Unwanted local effects of inhaled steroids include:

- Oral candidiasis (thrush)
- Dysphonia.

Combination LABA/ICS inhalers

There are a number of different combinations presented in a variety of inhaler devices, these include:

- Salmeterol + fluticasone, three strength combinations as a metered dose inhaler (MDI) and three strength combinations as a dry powder inhaler (DPI)
- Formoterol + budesonide, three strength combinations as a DPI
- Formoterol + beclometasone, one strength combination as a MDI
- Formoterol + fluticasone, three strength combinations as a MDI.

In general, these combination inhalers are used as regular preventative therapy with the dose adjusted, to achieve long-term control of asthma; a short-acting beta agonist inhaler being used for control of breakthrough symptoms. However, a budesonide 200 µg/formoterol 6 µg dry powder inhaler has been granted a licence for preventer (maintenance) and reliever use for asthma. Thus some asthmatics who are using a budesonide 200 µg/formoterol 6 µg inhaler may only need to have one inhaler. A budesonide 200 µg/formoterol 6 µg inhaler can only be used for relief of symptoms if also being used as a regular preventer. It is not licensed for use before exercise to prevent exercise-induced asthma; an additional short-acting beta$_2$ agonist should be used for this purpose.

Fluticasone 500 µg/salmeterol 50 µg dry powder inhaler and budesonide 400 µg/formoterol 12 µg dry powder inhaler, twice daily, are licensed for patients with COPD whose forced expiratory volume in 1 s (FEV$_1$) is less than 50–60% predicted and who are frequent exacerbators (two or more exacerbations per year).

The peak flow meter

The PFM is a simple inexpensive device, prescribable on the NHS, which gives a useful objective measure of airways obstruction. A PFM and its correct use is illustrated in Fig. 14.2. The PFM measures peak expiratory flow rate (PEFR). PEFR is expressed in litres per minute (L/min). Flow rate of gas through a tube is proportional to the diameter of the tube when the pressure exerted on the gas is constant. Thus the maximum rate at which individuals can expel air from their lungs is proportional to the patency of the tubes in their lungs. A reduced PEFR indicates that there is obstruction to airflow in the lungs.

Asthmatics will obtain useful information about their condition by using the PFM twice daily and charting their results for 2–4 weeks in the following situations:

- To confirm a diagnosis of asthma (a diurnal variation of PEFR of more than 20% is characteristic of asthma)

1 Set marker to zero
2 Stand up, hold PFM horizontally, avoiding touching or blocking the movement of the marker
3 Breathe in deeply then blow into the PFM as fast and hard as possible
4 Note reading, reset marker and repeat twice
5 The peak flow is the highest of the three readings

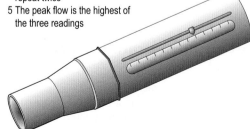

Fig. 14.2 The correct use of a peak flow meter (PFM).

- To establish the level of control of asthma on current therapy
- To track improvement of control of asthma following the introduction of a new treatment
- To ensure asthma control is maintained when treatment is stepped down
- As an aid to self-management of asthma.

Normal values are available for PEFR in graph or chart form or on 'wheels'. In adults, normal values for PEFR vary by age, sex and height; for children, PEFR varies just by height. Normal or average values of PEFR are just that and values of 50–100 L/min above or below a predicted value fall within the normal range. An increase of at least 20% in PEFR following the use of an inhaled short-acting beta$_2$ agonist such as salbutamol is diagnostic of asthma. This is known as a *reversibility test*.

The PFM is of less value in COPD as the airway obstruction tends to be fixed rather than variable, and lung volumes may be more important. Spirometry, which measures FEV$_1$ and forced vital capacity (FVC), is a more useful test of lung function in COPD.

Types of inhaler device

Aerosol inhalers

Metered dose inhaler

An MDI (Fig. 14.3) delivers an aerosol of drug dissolved or suspended in a propellant. Immediately an MDI is actuated, some of the propellant rapidly evaporates to produce droplets of appropriate size to be inhaled into the lung. Further evaporation of propellant may occur in the mouth and the so-called 'cold-freon effect' occurs if there is further evaporation of propellant (freon) when the aerosol impacts on the back of the throat. The sensation produced by the cold-freon effect can be sufficient in a minority of individuals to stop the inhalation and means that these individuals cannot use MDIs. The propellants currently used are generally hydrofluoroalkanes (HFAs). Chlorofluoroalkanes, also known as *chlorofluorocarbons (CFCs)*, were formerly used as propellants, but are now banned by international treaty because of their ozone-depleting properties. It should perhaps be noted that while HFAs do not have the ozone-depleting effects of CFCs, both CFCs and HFAs are 'greenhouse' gases.

Surfactants such as oleic acid and co-solvents such as ethanol may be used to facilitate the production of an appropriate suspension or solution of drug in propellant.

The propellants, which are gases at room temperature, are maintained as liquids by filling under pressure into the metal aerosol canister.

A metered dose is achieved by having an appropriate size reservoir in the valve, which fills by gravity as the valve re-seats after each actuation.

The correct method of using an MDI is shown in Fig. 14.4.

Common errors in using an MDI include:

- Inability to coordinate actuation of the inhaler with inspiration

**HOW TO USE A
METERED DOSE INHALER**

1 Shake the inhaler then remove cap
2 Breathe out slowly and gently
3 Place the mouthpiece in your mouth
4 When you start to breathe in, press down on the canister and continue to breathe in deeply and slowly
5 Hold your breath for 10–15 seconds
6 Remove the mouthpiece from your mouth, then breathe out
7 For a further dose, repeat steps 1 to 6 after a 30 second wait
8 Replace the cap and store in a cool place

A Metered Dose Inhaler

**ALWAYS DEMONSTRATE TO THE PATIENT HOW TO USE THE
METERED DOSE INHALER**

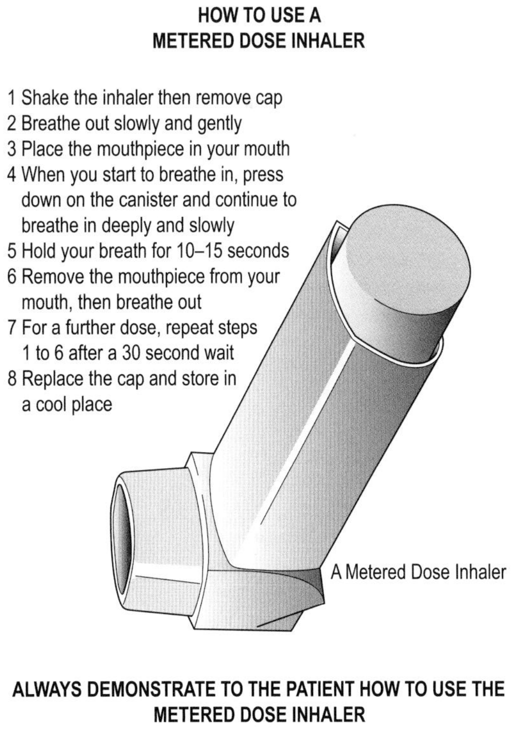

Fig. 14.4 How to use a metered dose inhaler. (*Source*: Education for Health.)

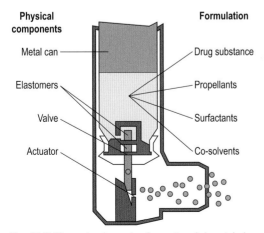

Fig. 14.3 The main elements of a metered dose inhaler.

Physical components — Formulation
Metal can — Drug substance
Elastomers — Propellants
Valve — Surfactants
Actuator — Co-solvents

- Taking a short, sharp inspiration, instead of a long, steady inspiration (this is often at least in part due to not exhaling before using the inhaler)
- Actuating the inhaler twice (or more) on one inspiration.

Breath-actuated MDI

Inhaling through a breath-actuated MDI triggers a mechanism that 'fires' (actuates) the aerosol. These inhalers are particularly useful for those patients who have difficulty coordinating inspiration with actuation of the MDI.

Easi-Breathe is a type of breath-actuated MDI; its correct use is shown in Fig. 14.5.

Autohaler is another breath-actuated MDI. Using an Autohaler is essentially the same as using an Easi-Breathe except that the Autohaler is primed by raising a lever on the top of the inhaler, whereas the Easi-Breathe is primed by opening the mouthpiece cover.

Common errors when using a breath-actuated MDI include:
- Not achieving a sufficiently high inspiratory flow rate to actuate the device
- Stopping inhaling immediately the inhaler actuates.

MDI + spacer

A chamber device (spacer) may be attached to an MDI (Fig. 14.6).

A spacer consists of a plastic chamber with a port at one end for the MDI and in most cases a one-way valve and mouthpiece at the other end.

An MDI + spacer is best used by firing a single dose from the MDI; inhalation should then start as soon as possible.

A spacer may be used with an MDI for the following reasons:
- To overcome difficulty in coordinating inspiration with actuation of the MDI, as the inspirable particles remain available for inhalation for some seconds after actuation
- To decrease deposition of non-respirable particles in the oropharynx. The larger particles are deposited in the spacer, rather than the oropharynx. This may be particularly important for high-dose inhaled steroids
- To allow those unable to distinguish between inspiration and expiration (e.g. young children) to benefit from inhaled therapy by simply inhaling and exhaling across the one-way valve

HOW TO USE THE EASI-BREATHE

1 Shake the inhaler then open the cap
2 Breathe out slowly and gently
3 Place the mouthpiece in your mouth and close your mouth tightly around it
4 Keeping the inhaler upright, breathe in slowly and deeply. Don't stop breathing in when the inhaler 'puffs'.
5 Hold your breathe for 10–15 seconds, then remove mouthpiece
6 For a further dose, repeat steps 1–5 after a 30 second wait
7 Replace cap and store in a cool place

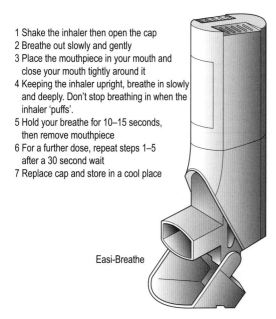

Easi-Breathe

ALWAYS DEMONSTRATE TO THE PATIENT HOW TO USE THE EASI-BREATHE

Fig. 14.5 How to use the Easi-Breathe. (*Source*: Education for Health.)

HOW TO USE A SPACER DEVICE
e.g. VOLUMATIC

Single breath technique

1 Shake the inhaler and remove the cap
2 Insert the inhaler into the device
3 Place the mouthpiece of the device into your mouth
4 To release a dose of the drug, press down once on the canister
5 Breathe in slowly and deeply
6 Hold your breath for about 10 seconds, then breathe out into the mouthpiece of the device
7 Breathe in again, then remove the mouthpiece from your mouth
8 For a further dose, repeat steps 1–7, after a 30 second wait

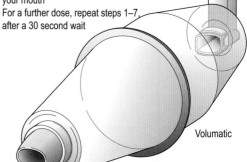

Volumatic

ALWAYS DEMONSTRATE TO THE PATIENT HOW TO USE THE SPACER DEVICE

Fig. 14.6 How to use a spacer device, e.g. Volumatic. Method for patients who can use the device without help. (*Source*: Education for Health.)

- To deliver a large dose of bronchodilator in an acute attack. Current guidelines advocate inhaling single doses serially. There has also been a practice of actuating a number of doses into the larger volume spacers (e.g. Volumatic) and then breathing tidally across the one-way valve.

A mask may be attached or be integral to a spacer. The mask can then be placed over the mouth and nose of babies or infants to enable them to benefit from inhaled therapy. The correct use of a spacer and face mask is shown in Fig. 14.7.

Examples of spacers are Volumatic, Nebuhaler and AeroChamber.

Dry powder inhaler

Medicines for inhalation can be presented as a micronized powder. The powder may be pure drug as in some Turbohalers, or be drug and a carrier powder such as lactose, as in Diskhaler and Accuhaler.

When a carrier powder is used, the drug particles are adhered by weak electrostatic forces to the much larger carrier particles. As the drug/carrier powder is inhaled from the inhaler, the small respirable drug particles fly off the larger non-respirable carrier particles. The lactose carrier thus remains in the mouth. Patients using DPIs that employ a carrier powder should be reassured that even when using the inhaler correctly, they will have carrier powder left in the mouth.

Patients inhaling pure drug from a Turbohaler providing only drug may experience little or no taste.

The correct method of using the Turbohaler is shown in Fig. 14.8 and the Accuhaler in Fig. 14.9.

All inhalers are boxed with instruction leaflets. However, the best way to learn how to use an inhaler is to have the technique demonstrated, then to attempt to use the inhaler under supervision, so that any errors can be corrected. Many patients will benefit from pharmacists providing this service. Similarly, for pharmacists to best learn how to provide this service, they too should be shown how to use the inhaler and how to spot common errors. Medical representatives from companies that market inhalers are usually more than happy to train pharmacists how to use, demonstrate and check

**HOW TO USE A LARGE-VOLUME
SPACER AND MASK**

1 Remove the mouthpiece cover from the inhaler
2 Attach the mask to the spacer mouthpiece
3 Shake the inhaler and insert into the spacer device
4 Tip the spacer to an angle of 45° or more to enable the
   valve to remain open
5 Apply the mask to the child's face covering nose and mouth
   with as tight a seal as possible
6 Press the inhaler canister once to release a dose of the medication,
   keep the mask on the child's face to allow 5 or 6 breaths
7 Wait for 30 seconds before repeating
8 When using this method to administer inhaled
   steroids, remember to wash the child's
   face after each treatment

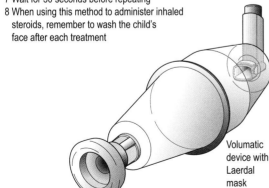

Volumatic
device with
Laerdal
mask

**ALWAYS DEMONSTRATE TO THE PATIENT HOW TO USE THE
LARGE-VOLUME SPACER AND MASK**

Fig. 14.7 How to use a large-volume spacer and face mask. *Source*: Education for Health.

HOW TO USE THE TURBOHALER

1 Remove the cap by unscrewing
2 Whilst holding the Turbohaler upright, twist the base clockwise
   then back again until a click is heard
3 Breathe out slowly and gently, then place mouthpiece between teeth
   and lips and breathe in deeply and slowly
4 Hold breathe for about 10 seconds, remove
   Turbohaler from mouth and then
   breathe out
5 Repeat steps 2 and 4, if another dose
   is required
6 Replace cap
7 Twenty doses are left when a red line
   shows in the window at the side of the
   Turbohaler. The Turbohaler is empty
   when the red line completely fills the
   window.

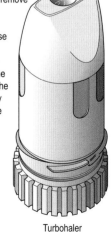

Turbohaler

**ALWAYS DEMONSTRATE TO THE PATIENT HOW TO USE THE
TURBOHALER**

Fig. 14.8 How to use the Turbohaler. *Source*: Education for Health.

111

HOW TO USE THE ACCUHALER

1 Open the outer case of the Accuhaler. Ask your pharmacist if unsure how to do this
2 With the mouthpiece facing you, slide the lever away from you until you hear a click. This procedure moves the dose counter on and makes the dose available
3 Breathe out slowly and gently, then place the mouthpiece between teeth and lips
4 Breathe in deeply and slowly
5 Remove the mouthpiece and hold breath for about 10 seconds
6 Repeat steps 2–5 for a second dose
7 Close the Accuhaler
8 The dose counter is red when 5 doses are left

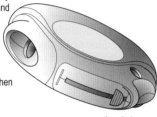

Accuhaler

ALWAYS DEMONSTRATE TO THE PATIENT HOW TO USE THE ACCUHALER

Fig. 14.9 How to use the Accuhaler. *Source*: Education for Health.

Table 14.1 Differences in the use and care of metered dose inhalers and dry powder inhalers

MDI	DPI
Coordination of actuation and inhalation required	No coordination required as the release of powder and inhalation is a two-step process
Long, slow inhalation is the ideal to allow vaporization of propellants	Inhalation should be vigorous to disperse drug particles
The outer plastic housing of the inhaler (aerosol canister removed) can be washed to prevent blockage of actuator	Inhalers containing drug, e.g. Turbohaler, must never be washed
Exhalation prior to inhalation can be into the inhaler	Exhalation must never be into the inhaler

inhaler technique. As part of this service, the medical representative will provide placebo inhalers, to allow the pharmacist to demonstrate the correct inhaler technique, instruction leaflets and other patient education material. Pharmacists can also signpost patients to demonstration videos on websites such as www.asthma.org.uk.

The use and care of a DPI differs from that of an MDI, as shown in Table 14.1.

Nebulizers

Medicines for inhalation can be presented as solutions or suspensions for nebulization. A nebulizing system (Fig. 14.10) usually consists of a compressor supplying compressed air to a nebulizing chamber, which delivers the nebulized drug to the patient via a mouthpiece or face mask. The face mask is most commonly used but when deposition of the nebulized drug on the face is undesirable (e.g. a steroid), then a mouthpiece is preferable, or the face under the mask should be protected with petroleum jelly. A mouthpiece is also needed with inhaled ipratropium to prevent the potential precipitation of closed angle glaucoma.

The principle of jet nebulization is shown in Fig. 14.11. The gas used to drive the nebulization process may be oxygen or air, but in either case a minimum flow rate of 8 L/min at a pressure of at least 69 kPa (10 psi) is required.

Patients using more than one nebulized medicine may have two different solutions mixed in the nebulizing chamber to be nebulized together. The summary of product characteristics (SPC) may give advice on other solutions and diluents that may be appropriately mixed with a given medicine for nebulization. It is possible that one solution will precipitate the other; this can normally be detected by the mixed solutions in the nebulizer chamber changing from clear to cloudy. Such a change means that the mixed solutions are not compatible and should not be nebulized together. Consideration should also be given to the total volume of the mixed solutions, as the larger the volume, the longer it will take to be nebulized.

Nebulizers are used when high doses of drug are required and/or when the patient is unable to use any form of inhaler. Nebulizers do not require the patient to learn any technique and are effective on normal or shallow breathing.

Nebulizers are used in the treatment of severe acute asthma and this is best done under medical supervision:
- To ensure that an adequate objective and maintained response to treatment is achieved (e.g. by measuring PEFR before and after nebulization)
- To assess if other treatment is indicated, e.g. oral or parenteral steroids
- To plan follow-up and possible review of chronic medication.

Nebulized treatment may also be used in the latter stages of COPD often in conjunction with domiciliary oxygen therapy. Domiciliary oxygen cylinders do not provide sufficient flow rates to produce adequate nebulization, so a compressor unit should be used.

Drugs for nebulization are normally presented as unit dose vials; examples of these are Nebules and Respules.

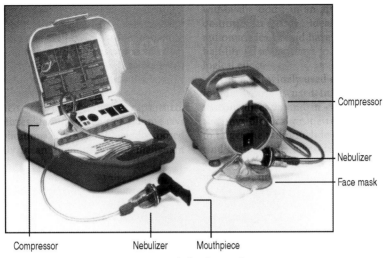

Fig. 14.10 Nebulization equipment.

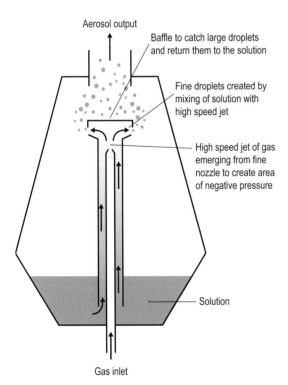

Aerosol output

Baffle to catch large droplets
and return them to the solution

Fine droplets created by
mixing of solution with
high speed jet

High speed jet of gas
emerging from fine
nozzle to create area
of negative pressure

Solution

Gas inlet

Fig. 14.11 The principle of jet nebulization.

Key points

- Asthma and COPD are common conditions, treatment of which is largely dependent on the inhaled route
- The vast majority of inhaled treatments for asthma and COPD can be divided into two pharmacological classes of drugs: inhaled bronchodilators and inhaled steroids
- Inhaled bronchodilators can be further subdivided into beta$_2$ agonists and muscarinic agonists. Each of these classes can be further subdivided into short acting and long acting
- National and international management guidelines are available for asthma and COPD and treatment is based on a step-wise approach
- A range of inhalation devices is available to deliver drugs directly to the lungs. This has clear advantages including using much lower doses compared with oral therapy
- The use of inhalers is technique dependent and patients require training in their use
- Medicines to be inhaled are presented as aerosol inhalers, dry powder inhalers or liquids to be nebulized
- The most widely prescribed inhaler device is the aerosol metered dose inhaler (MDI). The MDI may be used in conjunction with a spacing device (a 'spacer'). A modified form of the MDI, triggered to actuate by inhalation, is a breath-actuated MDI. Both the 'spacer' and the breath-actuated MDI overcome the main difficulty of using an MDI, the need to coordinate inhalation with actuation of the MDI, and allow a wider range of individuals to successfully use an MDI

- Dry powder inhalers (DPIs) were originally developed to overcome the difficulty some patients have coordinating inhalation with actuation of an MDI
- DPIs vary widely in appearance and the method by which the powder is made available for inhalation, but all rely on inhalation to mobilize the powder from the inhaler and through the mouthpiece
- Liquids for nebulization are either solutions or permanent suspensions. It may be that solutions are more reliably nebulized and inhaled than permanent suspensions
- Caution should be exercised when mixing two liquids for nebulization in the nebulizer, as one liquid can cause precipitation in the other

- The peak flow meter is a simple prescribable device which gives an objective measurement of lung function, and can be useful from time to time for asthmatics, e.g. when commencing a new treatment. It may also be used to aid self-management of asthma
- Many asthmatic and COPD patients will have at least two or three different inhalers. They will obtain greatest benefit from their inhalers if they understand something about their condition, the rationale for the different inhalers and how and when to use them
- Pharmacists with an understanding of asthma and COPD treatment and the correct use of inhalers can provide advice, education and training for patients on inhaled therapy, which can markedly improve patients' quality of life.

Chapter 15

Parenteral nutrition and dialysis

Lindsay Harper and Liz Lamerton

STUDY POINTS

- Provision of nutritional support for patients
- Indications for total parenteral nutrition (TPN)
- Components and compounding of a TPN/home parenteral nutrition (HPN) formulation
- Addition of medicines to a TPN or HPN bag
- HPN training and potential problems
- Administration of a TPN/HPN formulation
- British Parenteral Nutrition Group and British Association of Parenteral and Enteral Nutrition
- Introduction to home-care for patients on dialysis
- Haemodialysis (HD), peritoneal dialysis (PD), including continuous ambulatory peritoneal dialysis (CAPD), intermittent peritoneal dialysis (IPD) and automated peritoneal dialysis (APD)
- Dialysis solutions
- Provision of services from a hospital renal unit, including home dialysis

Introduction

Today, an increasing number of patients are requesting and being provided with healthcare services at home. Such services include the provision of home parenteral nutrition and home dialysis. This chapter will explore the provision of parenteral nutrition and dialysis for patients in hospital and will explain how these services can be transferred to the home-care setting.

Provision of nutritional support

Studies have shown that up to 50% of medical and surgical patients can suffer from nutritional deficiencies. If nutritional support is indicated, enteral feeding should be considered as the first option. Patients can receive nutrients orally or via a tube feed, e.g. by nasogastric feeding. This is only possible if the gastrointestinal tract is functional. If this is not the case, parenteral nutrition may be considered. Short-term (e.g. postoperative) intravenous (IV) administration of fluids, such as 5% dextrose or saline may be sufficient. This could provide the patient with around 500 calories per day but does not provide any protein, vitamins, minerals or trace elements.

Patients who need longer-term nutrition support may require total parenteral nutrition (TPN), which is a method of administering adequate nutrients via the parenteral route. The components of a TPN formulation are added to a sterile infusion bag and administered to the patient via a catheter. Administration can be via a peripheral Venflon, a peripherally inserted central catheter (PICC) or a central line. However, TPN fluids are normally highly concentrated mixtures, which on a long-term basis could cause damage to peripheral veins. For this reason, peripheral veins are only used for TPN administration lasting up to 4 weeks.

If parenteral nutrition is supplied to patients at home, it is known as *home parenteral nutrition (HPN)* and is more likely to be provided by a commercial company than a hospital TPN unit. Patients on HPN administer their nutrition via a central line into a central vein.

Parenteral nutrition formulations are prepared under strict aseptic conditions (see Ch. 11) following guidelines published by the MHRA in *Rules and Guidance for*

Pharmaceutical Manufacturers (2002) and by the DH in *Aseptic Dispensing for NHS Patients* (Farwell 1995).

HPN is becoming increasingly prevalent. Guidelines have been published by the British Association of Parenteral and Enteral Nutrition (BAPEN) and the National Institute for Health and Care Excellence (NICE) to ensure that adequate provision is made for patients receiving HPN. Patients who are suitable candidates for HPN will be, initially, stabilized on TPN bags while in hospital. They can then undergo appropriate training to enable them to administer their TPN bags at home. If the patient is unable to care for their line, then a carer or nurse would be trained to administer the TPN at home. However, HPN patients will still need to return to the hospital for regular check-ups. This means that pharmacists involved in the care of HPN patients will require a working knowledge of the procedures adopted to provide care for patients in hospital and at home. They may also have to liaise with the patient's GP and the community nurse.

This chapter concentrates on the provision of adult TPN, although neonatal TPN is available.

Indications for TPN

TPN can be required for finite periods of time or for life. Some of the main indications for TPN are:

- Gastrointestinal disease, including Crohn's disease, ulcerative colitis, pancreatitis and malabsorption syndrome
- Major trauma including severe burns, severe septicaemia
- Major abdominal surgery; severely malnourished patients may benefit from early peri- and postoperative parenteral nutrition if surgery has resulted in a non-functioning gastrointestinal tract
- Malignancy of the small bowel
- Radiation enteritis, when TPN is considered if enteritis is severe after treatment of a primary malignancy
- High-dose chemotherapy, radiotherapy and bone marrow transplantation. Patients are often ill for a limited time (3–6 weeks) and are unable to eat. TPN can be administered during this period to ensure that the patient's nutritional requirements are adequately met.

Several other conditions may require the nutritional support of TPN, e.g. patients in a prolonged coma or patients with AIDS.

Assessment of the patient in hospital

TPN aims to provide patients with all their nutritional requirements in one formulation, which can then be infused directly into the body via the veins, either central or peripheral. In order to determine exactly what the patient's nutritional requirements are, clinical and biochemical assessments must take place. The Malnutrition Universal Screening Tool (MUST) is used to identify patients who may benefit from TPN. The patient's body weight, height and body mass index (BMI) can be recorded and comparison made with their ideal body weight which would be available from standard charts. In most hospitals, a dietitian would review the patient and calculate their nutritional requirements.

Factors investigated will include urea and electrolytes, full blood counts, liver function tests, triglycerides, blood glucose and fluid balance. Trace elements are only monitored if the patient receives TPN for longer than 28 days. The NICE guidelines for nutrition support contain a section on the monitoring required for TPN patients.

Each hospital has its own particular way of designing a TPN regimen. Most hospitals use a range of standard formulations which are routinely used to treat TPN patients. Standard bags can be altered if the need arises. In general, additions to the finished TPN bags, outside of the pharmacy aseptic unit, are not recommended in order to minimize microbial contamination.

More recently, pharmaceutical companies have introduced a range of three-in-one ready-to-use multi-chambered TPN bags. These bags have three chambers, which contain amino acid, dextrose and lipid. When a bag of TPN is required, the seal separating the chambers can easily be broken and the three solutions are mixed together in one chamber. Before mixing, these bags have a long expiry date of around 2 years and do not need to be stored in the fridge. Many hospitals have swapped to using these bags as they are cost-effective and reduce the time for manufacture. Trace elements and vitamins need to be added to these bags before use.

Some hospitals tailor regimens to individual patients and carry out a number of calculations to determine baseline requirements for each component. In this way, they can build up a formulation by matching up the patient's requirements to commercially available solutions, which contain the required components in the correct proportions. Individualized bags tend to be used in patients on long-term TPN. Patients on HPN will always have bags tailored exactly to their nutritional needs.

The nutrition team

In most hospitals where TPN is supplied, there will be a nutrition team to coordinate the delivery of the parenteral nutrition service. This team can include the following:

- Consultant
- Senior registrar/registrar

- Pharmacist
- Clinical psychologist
- Nutrition nurse(s)
- Dietitian(s)
- Biochemist(s).

The role of these individuals in provision of patient care can vary from one hospital to another. In general, the consultant is responsible for prescribing the TPN formulation and liaising with the patient's GP to provide care for HPN patients although, with the introduction of non-medical prescribing, this role is increasingly taken over by nurses and pharmacists.

The pharmacist can provide information on aseptic techniques for handling and setting up TPN bags, formulation requirements, potential complications or stability problems, and storage conditions required. In some hospitals, the pharmacist's role can be extended to include the following:

- Training nursing staff in the techniques required for IV administration of TPN fluids
- Helping with patient training for HPN
- Monitoring of patients in HPN clinics
- Liaising with the staff from the home-care company
- Advising on the patient's drug therapy
- Liaising with the patient's community pharmacist.

The nutrition nurse and dietitian will together give advice on a day-to-day basis regarding the nutritional status of the patients and will advise on necessary dietary requirements.

Commercial companies supplying home-care services have a nutrition nurse who provides medical care, support and advice (on a 24-hour basis if required), a patient coordinator who deals with the ordering of HPN bags and ancillaries, and a designated delivery person who will supply the necessary equipment and HPN bags to the patient's home.

In the rare circumstances that the HPN is supplied by the hospital pharmacy, patients can be provided with the support from the hospital and their GP.

Components of a TPN formulation

TPN formulations can contain the following components:
- Water
- Protein source – measured in grams of nitrogen
- Energy source – carbohydrate and fat
- Electrolytes
- Trace elements
- Vitamins and minerals.

Baseline water requirements

Water accounts for over 50% of body weight. To prevent patients becoming dehydrated, daily water losses and gains must be carefully considered. Water can be lost through urine and faeces and through 'insensible losses', i.e. through the skin and lungs. Patients with burns and gastrointestinal losses will require increased volume. Patients with renal and cardiac failure should be given reduced volumes.

Several methods are available for estimating daily fluid requirements, but most take into consideration body weight and measured urine output, and an allowance is made for insensible losses. The average adult requires between 1500 and 4000 mL of fluid per day. A TPN regimen will need to provide this volume of fluid on a daily basis.

Protein source

Protein requirements vary from one patient to another and are highly dependent on the metabolic status of the patient. Undernourished patients requiring parenteral nutrition are, generally, said to have a negative nitrogen balance. This means that the amount of nitrogen excreted in urine and faeces is greater than the amount of nitrogen administered.

Lack of nitrogen in the body can result in poor wound healing and interference with the body's defence mechanisms. To overcome this problem, a utilizable source of nitrogen must be administered to the patient. This is achieved by administering amino acid solutions in a TPN formulation. Nitrogen requirements can be estimated from a 24-hour urine collection. This is done by analysing the total amount of urea excreted and by considering the individual patient's body weight and clinical 'type'.

Energy sources

Carbohydrates and fats are chosen to provide optimal energy sources for TPN patients. The relative proportions of each

---

Example 15.1

A postoperative surgical patient requires 0.2 g/kg/24 h of nitrogen. The patient weighs 47 kg.

$$\text{Nitrogen requirements per day} = 0.2 \times 47 \text{ kg}$$
$$= 9.4 \text{ g nitrogen}$$

This requirement can then be matched up to commercially available solutions. Each gram of amino acid nitrogen is equivalent to 6.25 g of protein, e.g. Vamin 9 contains 9.4 g of nitrogen per litre. This is equivalent to 60 g of protein and will provide the patient with the required daily nitrogen intake. However, care must also be taken when selecting an amino acid solution for inclusion in a TPN formulation, as most commercially available solutions are hypertonic in nature and have a pH between 5 and 7.4. The pH of the amino acid solution may have an effect on the overall stability of the formulation and must be considered carefully.

will be dependent on the clinical requirements of the patient and formulation considerations. The carbohydrate of choice is normally dextrose and is available in solution with concentrations ranging from 5% to 70% weight in volume (w/v). Like amino acid solutions, dextrose solutions are hypertonic and have a low pH (3–5). If high concentrations of dextrose are added to the TPN bags, they must only be given centrally.

The fat component in a TPN formulation is administered in the form of an oil-in-water emulsion. Fat emulsions are isotonic with plasma, have neutral pH and provide a high calorie source in a low volume. As a result, they are often used in combination with dextrose to provide the necessary calorie content, thereby avoiding the potential problems encountered with excessive dextrose administration.

Fat emulsions provide the patient with essential fatty acids and also act as a vehicle for fat-soluble vitamins, which are required in the TPN formulation. Fat is not required in every TPN formulation, but fat deficiency can occur in patients who do not receive fat components for periods longer than 1 month.

Commercially available preparations are based on soya bean oils and are composed of varying combinations of long and medium chain triglycerides. Newer fat solutions have been developed, incorporating olive oil and fish oils, which are claimed to protect patients on long-term parenteral nutrition from complications. Larger and longer trials are required to prove these claims. The energy content of commercially available solutions for both carbohydrates and fats is expressed in kcal/L, e.g. Intralipid 10% provides 550 kcal/500 mL; dextrose 5% provides 210 kcal/500 mL.

Electrolytes

The main electrolytes of clinical significance in a TPN formulation include sodium, potassium, magnesium, calcium, phosphate and chloride. The requirement for electrolytes can be met in the form of injectable solutions of varying percentage content. Electrolyte content of each is expressed in terms of mmol/L. The individual role of each electrolyte in a TPN formulation is given in Table 15.1.

Trace elements

Trace elements act as metabolic cofactors and are said to be essential for the proper functioning of several enzyme systems in the body. Despite being termed *essential*, they are only required in very small quantities, expressed in micromoles. The main trace elements required in a TPN formulation are zinc, copper, manganese and chromium.

Vitamins and minerals

Vitamin requirements fall into two categories: fat soluble and water soluble. Four fat-soluble vitamins (vitamins A,

D, E and K) and nine water-soluble vitamins (vitamins B_1, B_2, B_3, B_5, B_6, B_{12}, C, folic acid and biotin) are said to be essential.

Vitamins and minerals are normally included in foods taken in orally and must therefore be included in TPN formulations for patients on long-term parenteral nutrition. The NICE guidelines published in 2006 recommend that patients must receive vitamins and trace elements daily in their TPN bags.

Compounding of TPN and HPN formulations

Compounding can take place within a hospital pharmacy using aseptic dispensing facilities within a clean room or within a designated compounding unit in a commercial pharmaceutical company.

Preparation and training

For patients in hospital, a suitable TPN regimen will be prescribed. On receipt of the prescription, the pharmacist checks the suitability and compatibility of the formulation, the required volume of each component is calculated and details are transferred to a worksheet. Patient details are entered into a computer and labels generated for the worksheet and the final product. In the preparation area, items required for the compounding process are collected together in an appropriate tray, ready for transfer to the clean room facility. Batch numbers and expiry dates for each product used are recorded on the worksheet. The pharmacist checks all details, including calculations, before the compounding procedure begins.

Compounding of a TPN formulation is carried out under strict aseptic conditions (in a Grade A environment) using a laminar airflow (LAF) cabinet within a clean room facility. Chapter 11 gives details regarding clean room facilities, gowning-up procedures for entry to clean rooms, and working procedures for using LAF cabinets. Standard operating procedures (SOPs) should be available for all staff carrying out aseptic dispensing procedures.

TPN/HPN bags

The components of a TPN formulation are sterile, and are prepared under sterile conditions, as the formulation is eventually infused directly into the bloodstream of the patient. It is therefore essential that the bags used to hold the TPN formulation are also sterile. In the past, only polyvinyl chloride (PVC) bags were used for TPN formulations. However, because of the problems of leaching of plasticizers from PVC bags containing a fat component, ethylvinyl

Table 15.1 Role of electrolytes used in TPN formulations

Electrolyte	Principal function	Daily intravenous requirement	Symptoms of deficiency	Symptoms of excess	Common sources
Sodium	Main extracellular cation Regulation of water balance Neuromuscular contractility	1–2 mmol/kg	Weakness, lethargy, confusion, convulsions, appetite, nausea and vomiting	Lethargy, coma, convulsions, muscle rigidity, thirst	Sodium chloride Sodium acetate Sodium phosphate
Potassium	Main intracellular cation Regulation of acid–base balance	1–2 mmol/kg	Muscle weakness, ileus, arrhythmias, alkalosis	Muscle weakness, paraesthesia, bradycardia, nausea and vomiting	Potassium chloride Potassium phosphate
	Neuromuscular contractility				
Magnesium	Co-factor for enzyme systems Neuromuscular contractility	0.1–0.2 mmol/kg	Lethargy, cramps, tetany, paraesthesia, arrhythmias, excitability, hypokalaemia, hypocalcaemia	Decreased muscular activity, lethargy, depression	Magnesium sulphate Magnesium chloride
Calcium	Mineralization: bones + teeth Neuromuscular contractility	0.1–0.15 mmol/kg	Paraesthesia, tetany, fitting, confusion, arrhythmias	Nausea, anorexia, lethargy, muscle weakness, confusion	Calcium gluconate Calcium chloride
Phosphate	Main intracellular anion Acid–base balance Energy	0.5–0.7 mmol/kg	Weakness, tingling	Non-specific effects on calcium balance	Phosphate salts of sodium and potassium, hydrogen
Chloride	Main extracellular anion	1–2 mmol/kg	Alkalosis	Acidosis	Chloride salts of above cations
	Acid–base balance				

From Walker and Edwards 2003, reproduced by permission.

acetate (EVA) bags (which contain no plasticizers) are now recommended. However, EVA bags have been shown to be permeable to oxygen; hence multilayer EVA bags are now available for formulations requiring prolonged storage.

Bags are usually supplied with a pre-mounted sterile filling set attached. The filling set consists of a number of hollow plastic tubes (up to six), with a plastic spike attached to the end of each. The spikes are used to pierce the rubber septum of the bottles and bags of amino acids, glucose and fat emulsion, to enable filling of the components into the TPN bag. Clamps fitted with air vents are attached to each filling tube to clamp off the source bottles and bags when they are empty. Filling sets are used for compounding purposes only and are disconnected and replaced with a sterile hub before being sent out to the patient. Every HPN bag is supplied with a sterile giving set which allows the bag to be infused into the patient.

TPN bags vary in size, ranging from small 250 mL bags, used for neonatal TPN, up to 4 L bags for adult TPN. Fig. 15.1 shows a TPN bag with filling set attached.

Addition of components to a TPN bag

Components are added into the TPN bag in a strictly defined procedure. Small-volume additives can be added directly into large-volume fluids (but not directly into the fat component), or directly into the additive port on the bag (depending on manufacturers' recommendations). Amino acid solutions and glucose are added into the bag first, followed by any fat emulsion if required. To prevent precipitation of vitamins, they are, generally, only added immediately before administration.

Filling of the TPN bags can be achieved under gravity. The bag is placed on the floor of the LAF cabinet and

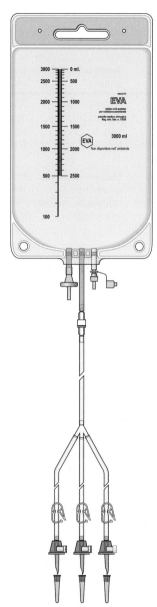

Fig. 15.1 A total parenteral nutrition (TPN) bag with filling set attached.

When all the components are added, the bag can be clamped off and the filling set removed. The bag is gently shaken to ensure adequate mixing of all components. The TPN bag and compounding materials are transferred back to the preparation area. A visual inspection of the bag is made, including checking of the additive port, for integrity. All necessary documentation is completed and the TPN bag is labelled. Details to be included on the label are shown in Box 15.1.

The TPN bag is then sealed into a dark-coloured outer plastic bag (to protect the formulation from light), and an outer label that is identical to the label on the bag itself is attached.

To maintain stability of the formulated product, it is refrigerated until required. All TPN and HPN formulations must be stored in a designated pharmaceutical grade refrigerator. Coolboxes, packed with ice packs, can be used for transportation of formulations to the ward or the patient's home.

Compounding of HPN formulations by commercial companies

A designated compounding unit is used for preparing HPN formulations. Conditions used will be the same as those used in the hospital sector, and the same government regulations apply. The compounding unit must hold a manufacturing licence prior to supplying TPN bags.

The commercial company providing the home-care service must be in receipt of a prescription for the HPN formulation prior to compounding.

However, when the health care is transferred to the home-care setting in Scotland, the patient's GP will take on the responsibility for supplying the HPN prescription. In England and Wales, the primary care commissioner is responsible for providing the HPN prescription, although with the current changes to the NHS in England and Wales the responsibilities may change. Subsequent prescriptions will then be forwarded to the commercial company in

the solution components suspended from a retort stand, enabling the solution to flow freely into the bag. If several bags require to be compounded in a limited time period, the bag can be placed in a vacuum chamber to speed up the filling process. Electronic devices, known as *compounders*, are also available. They are usually under microprocessor control, and can be pre-programmed to fill TPN bags with set volumes of individual components.

advance of the patient's requirements. The hospital nutrition team will issue the prescriptions for the patients at home. The patient coordinator will deal with orders for sundries and ancillaries such as pumps, dressings, needles, etc.

Potential complications arising during compounding and administration of TPN formulations

The components of a TPN formulation will individually and collectively contribute to the overall stability of the resulting formulation. However, with several hospitals now using standard TPN formulations, many of these problems can be overcome. For hospital pharmacies, which have a manufacturing licence, standard bags can be made up in advance of requirements and stored in a refrigerator for periods of 30 days or more. The shelf-life given to individual formulations must be based on validated stability studies previously carried out on the formulation. The stability of any regimen will be confirmed before manufacture.

Individual components of the formulation such as vitamins, electrolytes, and fat can cause formulation complications. Vitamin stability is very poor, particularly in the presence of light and with extended storage time. Stability is also affected by solution pH, hence the need for careful consideration of the overall formulation.

The requirement for administration of calcium and phosphate in a formulation can lead to precipitation of calcium phosphate. This reaction is said to be affected by factors such as the relative amounts of each component present, solution pH, concentration of amino acid solutions present and the mixing process used. To overcome this type of problem, manufacturers of parenteral nutrition fluids can supply tables, which give details of the amount of each component that can be safely combined to ensure stability of the formulation is maintained. These tables are specific to an individual formulation and details cannot be interchanged between formulations.

The presence of fat in a TPN formulation can cause stability problems. As storage time increases, the fat component of the formulation becomes less stable, resulting in a process of 'cracking' where the oil and water phases of the emulsion separate out. If the formulation is administered to the patient in this unstable condition, this can lead to potentially dangerous fat deposits arising in the lungs and other body tissues.

The factors a pharmacist must consider when formulating a TPN bag with a fat component are:
- The order in which components are added to the bag
- The types and amount of electrolytes present and their relative proportions – divalent and trivalent cations reduce stability

- The pH of the resultant mixture – higher pH improves stability
- Conditions arising during storage and administration
- The type of plastic bag used – EVA bags preferred.

Addition of medicines to a TPN or HPN bag

Stability studies have been carried out on a number of medicines to determine their compatibility and stability in a TPN bag. So far, studies have confirmed the suitability of only a limited range of medicines which includes: heparin, insulin, aminophylline, cimetidine, famotidine, ranitidine and certain antibiotics. Reference to manufacturers' literature and compatibility studies will provide current recommendations. Although stability is available on the drugs listed above, the addition of drugs to TPN is not recommended. This is because the drugs may affect the long-term stability of the TPN bag and it will affect the pharmacokinetics of the drugs added to the TPN. Most hospitals in the UK allow no additions to the TPN bags.

Administration of TPN/HPN formulations

For patients requiring TPN for longer than 4 weeks, central venous access is required. During their stay in hospital, patients have a catheter inserted into the subclavian vein under anaesthesia. It has an exit site on the lower chest wall, allowing patients easy access for care of the catheter site.

Catheters can be made of materials such as PVC or silicone. For long-term feeding, a permanent catheter (a Hickman catheter or a Portacath) is used. It is held in place by a Dacron cuff (an internal woven plastic used to connect arteries and veins under the skin). Good aseptic techniques are essential to ensure that the catheter site does not become contaminated. Infection around the catheter site can be difficult to treat successfully, and may eventually result in removal of the catheter and replacement at another site.

Catheter sites should only be used for administration of TPN fluids and not for blood sampling or administration of other medicines. In some instances, a triple lumen catheter can be used with one line being kept for administration of the TPN bag only. To infuse the TPN formulation into the patient, the catheter is connected via an extension set to a volumetric infusion pump. These devices use positive pressure as the driving force to allow accurate infusion at pre-set rates (see Ch. 12).

The infusion period varies from 24 h in hospital to around 12–14 h for home patients (as HPN can often be administered overnight). Most pumps now have the ability to be programmed to give an infusion rate which 'steps up' at the beginning and 'steps down' at the end of the infusion period, avoiding potential problems with high concentrations of dextrose in the formulation. They are also fitted with an alarm which will alert the patient if a technical fault arises.

Potential problems for HPN patients

Mechanical problems

Problems of pneumothorax, or air embolism, are more likely to occur in the hospital environment in the early stages of catheter placement, and are dealt with before the patient commences on HPN. However, daily connection and disconnection of the catheter hub may result in cracking and possible leakage of the HPN fluid. Repair kits are available, and if used promptly, when the problem first arises, catheter replacement may not be necessary.

Internal line blockage of the catheter can arise. Patients are taught to flush out the catheter port with heparinized saline to prevent thrombus formation. Blockage of the line arising during administration of the HPN fluid can cause changes in flow rate, which are recognized by the pump, and the alarm is activated.

Metabolic problems

Metabolic complications include:
- Problems with electrolyte levels leading to conditions such as hypernatraemia or hyponatraemia
- Problems with glucose levels leading to hyperglycaemia or hypoglycaemia
- Balancing of fluid intake (to ensure adequate hydration is achieved)
- Altered liver enzymes which can be resolved by amending the TPN prescription
- Metabolic bone disease, monitored by regular bone scans.

The majority of the metabolic complications which can affect HPN patients can be overcome by careful monitoring of the patient initially in hospital and with regular check-ups and home visits by the nutrition nurse.

Catheter-related complications

Catheter-related infections can arise as a result of poor management of the catheter exit site. Infection is distinguished by pain, redness and tenderness around the site and rigors when feeding through the line. To minimize such infections, staff are trained to use strict aseptic procedures when changing TPN bags and use of the catheter port is restricted to administration of the TPN bag only. HPN patients are taught the same aseptic techniques and are required to carry out these procedures at all times when changing bags at home. Home-care patients are also taught to be aware of their own physical condition and to be alert to any deterioration in their medical condition at the earliest possible time. Patients are asked to contact their nutrition nurse if they experience any signs or symptoms of infection around the catheter site.

Psychological and social problems

Patients receiving TPN in hospital, or at home, must learn to adapt to the changes occurring in their lifestyle. Some patients have, over a prolonged period of time, suffered from a general deterioration in their health, and as a result adapt well to the initiation of parenteral nutrition as it improves their quality of life. Other patients require TPN as a result of major trauma, and these patients find the dramatic changes in their lifestyle very difficult to cope with.

While in the hospital receiving treatment, patients have the constant support of medical and nursing staff to help them to cope with any practical difficulties encountered. The clinical psychologist will review many patients before discharge and coping strategies will be discussed. The ability of patients to adapt to HPN is highly dependent on a number of factors:
- Patient's underlying medical condition
- Physical ability and capability of the patient
- Training and counselling prior to leaving hospital
- Home circumstances, particularly support from family members and the patient's GP
- Ability to deal with physical and emotional changes in lifestyle, e.g. dependence on others.
- Disruption to normal sleeping pattern during administration of the HPN bag overnight, and loss of 'social' eating can be difficult for many patients, particularly in the initial stages of HPN.

To enable a smooth transition from hospital to home to be achieved, patients require the services of the nutrition nurse and other healthcare workers to teach them the necessary skills required for handling, setting up their HPN bags and disconnecting them once the procedure is complete.

Training for HPN patients

Health care which can be provided at home has a number of advantages. Patients have a better quality of life and can become more independent as their confidence in providing self-care increases. However, motivation and confidence to carry out the required manipulations at home are essential. Thus training in the hospital environment is required to build up the necessary skills and techniques.

A discharge plan is required for each patient working towards home-care. BAPEN, a registered charity formed in 1992, has laid down guidelines for the provision of nutritional care at home. Individual hospitals will develop their own guidelines based on the advice given by BAPEN. The scope of BAPEN includes guidelines on the following matters:

- Details that should be included in a patient discharge plan
- Knowledge and practical skills which must be achieved by patients prior to discharge
- Guidelines for GPs on the provision of HPN
- Advice on how to liaise with the patient's GP to ensure that everyone is aware of their responsibilities
- Information regarding the supplier of the HPN bags and equipment and how this service will be provided
- Details of appropriate people who patients can contact for advice and help with any problems they have.

The length of time required for training can vary depending on the patient's underlying medical condition and personal approach to training. Patients must be taught aseptic techniques and the importance of ensuring that they are carried out correctly. They must demonstrate their skills and competence on several occasions prior to leaving the hospital. Areas covered during the training period include:

- Aseptic techniques for setting up and disconnecting the HPN bag
- Care of the catheter site
- How to deal with problems of the catheter blocking
- Setting the pump for infusion of the HPN bag
- Dealing with simple mechanical problems with the pump.

Information booklets on HPN and educational videos can be used with patients to reinforce the training received in hospital.

Services provided by home-care companies

Patients receiving home care will require certain practical arrangements to be put in place before HPN can be initiated. Home-care companies who provide services to HPN patients normally provide the following items for patient use: a refrigerator for storing HPN bags; a trolley for patients to set up their HPN bags aseptically; a drip stand and an infusion pump. Patients are required to have adequate storage space to keep any extra components which may be required for HPN administration and easy access to hand washing facilities for use prior to setting up their HPN bag. A home assessment will be completed by the home-care company and a nutrition nurse from the hospital before discharge to ensure the patient's home circumstances are suitable for HPN.

Support services provided for HPN patients

Patients will be metabolically stable prior to transfer to the home-care setting, hence frequency of monitoring will be reduced to a minimum. Patients can have monthly check-ups at the hospital initially, reducing to 3-monthly as they adapt to life on HPN. During visits, patients may be seen by the multidisciplinary nutrition team and reviewed by each member of the team. The pharmacist on the team will arrange any changes in the patient's TPN prescription. Routine monitoring can be carried out during these visits, including the following:

- Checking the patient's underlying medical condition
- Reviewing the patient's nutritional status, particularly in relation to their weight
- Routine haematological and biochemical tests
- Checking for any complications
- Reviewing the patient's psychological state.

The nutrition nurse will make home visits, if required, to check on aseptic techniques and any practical difficulties being encountered by patients and/or their partner or carer.

Patients on HPN can benefit from the support of others undergoing nutrition therapy at home. This is made possible by an organization called 'PINNT' (Patients on Intravenous and Nasogastric Nutrition Therapy). This charitable organization aims to support and bring together people who have similar medical conditions and could benefit from the moral support of others who understand the problems they face. PINNT provides practical help in areas such as provision of portable equipment for people on HPN who wish to go on holiday, help with holiday arrangements, including appropriate travel insurance and general advice on benefits available to HPN patients. A newsletter is produced on a regular basis and close links are kept between PINNT and BAPEN to ensure that patient needs are adequately met.

The British Parenteral Nutrition Group

Pharmacists in the UK can keep up-to-date with the working of organizations like PINNT and BAPEN by joining the British Parenteral Nutrition Group (BPNG). Currently, BPNG has a large membership, most of whom are hospital pharmacists working in the NHS. However, membership also includes dietitians, nutrition nurses, research workers, and members of commercial companies who work in the field of TPN and HPN. The BPNG exists to further the practice of TPN through a number of activities including research, contributing to the work of BAPEN and arranging symposia on practical and scientific developments in the field. This group is also one of five constituent groups which make up BAPEN.

Introduction to kidney disease and dialysis therapy

In December 2010 there were over 50,000 adult patients receiving renal replacement therapy in the UK. Patients requiring renal replacement therapy (RRT) have end-stage renal disease/failure (ESRF) which may have occurred acutely or may be the result of chronic kidney disease. Transplantation is the most common treatment modality (48%), with haemodialysis accounting for 44%, and peritoneal dialysis 8%, of RRT. Home therapies make up 9% of RRT. Home therapy was used by 17.6% of prevalent dialysis patients in 2010, with 2.9% on home haemodialysis, and the remaining patients having either continuous ambulatory peritoneal dialysis or automated peritoneal dialysis. While still small in number, more patients are now receiving home haemodialysis, with numbers increasing by 23% since 2009, from 636 patients to 780 patients.

Chronic kidney disease

Chronic kidney disease (CKD) is relatively common, affecting approximately 1 in 10 people in the general population. The most common cause is diabetes. Glomerulonephritis and hypertension are also responsible and less common causes include pyelonephritis. CKD may also be inherited, e.g. polycystic kidney disease. Some common drug therapies may also lead to kidney disease.

ESRF is the result of progressive kidney disease, which leads to an irreversible and life-threatening loss of function. Patients with ESRF may be suitable for RRT, or may choose conservative treatment. There are a number of types of RRT, e.g. kidney transplantation, haemodialysis or peritoneal dialysis. Unfortunately, over 30% of patients are unsuitable for transplantation and for a number of patients a suitable donor may not be found. For these patients, transplantation may not therefore be an option, and chronic RRT is required. For most patients with ESRF who wish to have RRT, there are two choices, either long-term haemodialysis (HD) or peritoneal dialysis (PD) therapy, although patients may not be suitable for both modalities and may change from one to the other at various times, according to need.

RRT with dialysis replaces only some of the functions of the kidneys and is an artificial method of filtering toxins and breakdown products from the blood. It does not replicate normal renal function, and does not provide any of the metabolic functions of the kidney, such as insulin metabolism or the hormonal functions, such as erythropoietin production. RRT with HD or PD uses a combination of dialysis therapy to remove unwanted solutes by the process of diffusion, and haemofiltration, and ultrafiltration to remove water.

Epidemiology

In 2010 the incidence rate in the UK was 107 per million population. The median age of all incident patients was 64.9 years and for non-whites 57.1 years. Diabetic renal disease is identified as the single most common cause in 24% of patients. There is no identified relationship between social deprivation and presentation pattern according to the renal registry data.

Dialysis

Dialysis is commenced to treat, or to prevent, life-threatening hyperkalaemia, acidosis or hypervolaemic pulmonary oedema, or to treat complications of CKD, e.g. pericarditis, uraemic neuropathy or seizures.

Haemodialysis

HD is a process where blood is filtered to remove waste products. The patient is connected to a dialysis machine where blood is removed from the patient's body and filtered by passing it over an artificial, semi-permeable membrane, into dialysis fluid. The waste products are retained within the dialysis fluid and the blood returned into the body.

To facilitate HD, access to the patient's bloodstream must be established, either using a surgically created arteriovenous fistula, where an artery is joined to a vein during a minor surgical operation, a graft, and the join between the artery and vein is made using a synthetic tube, or by inserting a permanent or temporary central vascular catheter into a large vein, such as the subclavian, jugular, or femoral vein.

HD usually takes 3–4 hours each time and will be required, on average, 3 times a week for most patients. The blood is removed, and passed over a membrane with a large surface area, to allow solutes to be exchanged between the blood and dialysis fluid. Dialysis membranes are sterile, disposable membranes made of cellulose or polycarbonate materials. Pressure is applied to the blood in the machine to induce an ultrafiltration process, and allow removal of excess water in addition to the removal of toxins.

Dialysis fluid is composed of similar constituents to plasma:

- Sodium
- Potassium
- Chloride
- Calcium
- Magnesium
- Glucose
- Bicarbonate, citrate, or lactate is added to buffer the solution.

To promote potassium removal from the blood, the dialysate potassium concentration is variable and is usually lower than that in the plasma. To prevent the blood clotting in the dialysis circuit, unfractionated heparin, low molecular weight heparin or prostacyclin may be used.

During the HD process, there are a number of potential complications, such as low blood pressure, air embolus and blood loss.

HD may be carried out in a variety of settings providing the appropriate equipment and water supply is available. Locations include specialist hospital units or in the patient's own home. The dialysis process follows the same principles in all settings.

Hospital-based haemodialysis

Patients occasionally have direct responsibility for their treatment; however, it is more common for the dialysis to be managed by a team of doctors, nurses, and other healthcare professionals. Patients travel to the unit for HD according to an arranged schedule.

In a satellite unit, patients sometimes play a more active role in their treatment. They are supervised by trained staff, but may prepare the dialysis machine or carry out the dialysis process themselves.

Home haemodialysis

Home HD may be suitable for a limited number of patients. NICE (TAC 48) recommends that all suitable patients should be offered home HD.

There are a number of advantages to home HD:

- Greater independence for the patient
- Excellent long-term outcome
- Improved blood pressure control
- Lower hospital admission rates
- Fewer limitations on timing of dialysis
- Greater flexibility
- No transport difficulties
- Optimal use of resources.

There are a number of factors that determine a patient's suitability for home HD. For example, patients must be able and motivated to learn and perform dialysis at home, and be capable of maintaining and monitoring their own treatment observations. They must be medically stable, and be free of complications that make dialysis difficult. Patients also require good functioning vascular access, support from family or carers and suitable space and facilities must be available. Any patients considered suitable for home HD will be assessed, including their home circumstances. They will undergo a comprehensive training programme to develop skills and techniques in addition to developing confidence and self-reliance.

Peritoneal dialysis

In PD, the dialysis fluid is passed directly into the patient's body and, in contrast to HD, no blood removal occurs. The peritoneal membrane which lines the abdominal cavity has a large surface area and a good capillary blood supply. It is this semi-permeable membrane that is used to perform PD, and allows excess water and waste products to be removed from the blood.

Dialysis fluid is instilled into the peritoneal cavity through a surgically inserted indwelling catheter, which goes through the abdominal wall. The distal end of the catheter has tiny holes in it to allow the dialysis fluid to flow freely into the peritoneal cavity. Fluid is removed from the blood by ultrafiltration down an osmotic pressure gradient. Solutes and toxins cross the peritoneal membrane through diffusion and solvent drag with water.

There are two main methods of PD: CAPD and APD.

In CAPD, patients generally carry out three or four PD exchanges every 24 h and this is the most common form of home dialysis. In APD, patients are connected to a machine for 8–12 h, often overnight. The machine utilizes a pump delivery system which warms the dialysis fluid prior to administration and delivers a carefully programmed volume of dialysis fluid which exchanges throughout the infusion period. The home patient or a carer will set the machine every night by connecting it to the catheter. This method of dialysis has advantages for the patient as it allows freedom from dialysis during the day.

A variety of dialysis fluids are available and each patient will be prescribed a specific tailored regimen of dialysis fluids. The volume will be determined in part by the available abdominal space. For adults, the range is 1–7 L.

The composition of the dialysate consists of sodium, calcium, glucose or dextran to increase or decrease osmolality.

The dialysis exchange requires strict aseptic technique and a number of different systems may be employed. The most popular is a disconnect system. Dialysis fluid is warmed to body temperature and both this and a drainage bag are attached to the abdominal catheter. Fluid is drained out from the abdominal catheter into the empty bag and new dialysate is instilled from the warmed bag. The bags are then disconnected and the fluid left in place for 4–8 h. The dialysate in the abdominal cavity drains in and out under gravity and by capillary blood flow.

The advantages of PD include the following:

- Independence – as the dialysis does not require hospital attendance or complex plumbing or machinery
- Continuous dialysis process is preferable, as the haemodynamic fluctuations are minimized
- Blood loss is avoided compared with HD, resulting in less anaemia
- Cost savings compared with HD
- Less fluid and dietary restriction.
  Disadvantages include:
- Infections of the peritoneum
- Glucose absorption from the dialysate
- Protein loss
- Treatment failure if the peritoneum is damaged.

Community dialysis teams

Community dialysis teams provide support to patients undertaking dialysis at home – both HD and PD. Most teams are multidisciplinary, with highly trained medical and nursing staff making decisions regarding the treatment and providing the care and support through regular home visits to monitor patients. The team will usually have strong links with the wider multidisciplinary team, which includes dietitians, pharmacists, renal technicians, and social workers.

Each member of the renal team will have specific responsibilities:

- The medical and nursing team will be involved with prescribing of dialysis programmes and clinical monitoring
- The dietitian advises on nutritional intake and any dietary restrictions required
- The pharmacist provides medicines advice and may have a role in the ordering and supply of dialysis fluids and ancillary products
- The social worker provides advice and practical help for patients
- The renal technician is responsible for the programming, servicing and functioning of dialysis machines.

UK Renal Pharmacy Group

The UK Renal Pharmacy Group (UKRPG) is affiliated to the British Renal Society, and is a specialist interest group for pharmacists and pharmacy technicians working in the field of renal medicine, or with an interest in renal pharmacy. The UKRPG uses its clinical pharmacy experience to compile *The Renal Drug Handbook* and *Introduction to Renal Therapeutics*; both publications are excellent reference sources for further reading.

Key points

- Up to half of medical and surgical patients may have nutritional deficiencies
- TPN/HPN formulations are prepared under strict aseptic conditions
- Before starting TPN, a full assessment of the patient's nutritional needs must be made
- The nutrition team contribute their expertise to provide good patient care by meeting regularly to monitor patient needs
- A TPN formulation may contain water, protein, carbohydrate, fat, electrolytes, trace elements, vitamins and minerals
- Most TPN patients have a negative nitrogen balance and so require amino acids
- Care must be taken when administering dextrose in a TPN/HPN formulation to prevent problems of hyper- or hypoglycaemia
- Strictly defined procedures are followed when adding ingredients to TPN bags during preparation
- Stability of TPN formulations is one of the major issues which must be carefully considered
- Controlling quantities can minimize incompatibilities such as that between calcium and phosphate
- TPN bags containing a fat component become less stable on prolonged storage, and could result in fat deposits arising in lungs and capillaries, if administered in this unstable condition
- For TPN lasting longer than 4 weeks, a central vein should be used
- A number of problems can arise during TPN/HPN administration. For HPN patients, adequate training to deal with problems arising at home is essential
- HPN patients are required to make psychological and social adjustments, but can also have an improvement in quality of life
- BAPEN has laid down standards for home nutritional care, which are used as the basis for patient training prior to discharge
- Dialysis is used to remove toxic metabolites, correct acid–base balance and avoid fluid overload
- In haemodialysis, the patient's blood is passed over a semi-permeable membrane to allow exchange of small solutes with dialysis fluid

- Peritoneal dialysis uses the peritoneal membrane as the semi-permeable membrane, the dialysis fluid staying in the peritoneal cavity during the exchange
- CAPD has a number of advantages and disadvantages for patients

- HD solutions do not need to be sterile, but PD solutions must be sterile and aseptic technique used in handling
- Home dialysis patients will require training and support

Chapter 16

Radiopharmacy

David Graham

STUDY POINTS

- Types of radionuclides and the principles of their medical use
- Examples of alpha-emitters, beta⁻- and beta⁺-emitters, electron capture and isomeric transitions
- Radionuclide production of beta⁺-emitters
- Principles of using a molybdenum-technetium generator
- Preparation of ^{99m}Tc radiopharmaceuticals
- Safety in radiopharmacy

Introduction

Elements that emit radiation are known as *radionuclides* and have a number of applications in medicine. Radiopharmacy in hospital practice is concerned with the manufacture or preparation of radioactive medicines known as *radiopharmaceuticals*. These have two main applications in medicine:

- As an aid to the diagnosis of disease (diagnostic radiopharmaceuticals)
- In the treatment of disease (therapeutic radiopharmaceuticals).

Diagnostic radiopharmaceuticals may be classified into two types:

- Radiopharmaceuticals used in tracer techniques for measuring physiological parameters (e.g. ^{51}Cr-EDTA for measuring glomerular filtration rate)
- Radiopharmaceuticals for diagnostic imaging (e.g. ^{99m}Tc-methylene diphosphonate (MDP) used in bone scanning).

In diagnostic imaging, gamma-emitting radionuclides are used, since their interaction with tissue is much less than that of particulate emitters and will cause significantly less damage to tissue. Radiopharmaceuticals are administered to the patient, usually by the intravenous (IV) route,

and distributed into a particular organ. The radiation is then detected externally using a special scintillation detector known as a *gamma-camera*. These are used by nuclear medicine departments to image the distribution of the radiopharmaceutical within the patient's body. Using the gamma-camera in conjunction with a computer system, it is not only possible to produce static images of an organ, but also to examine how the radiopharmaceutical moves through an organ. These dynamic images describe how the organ is functioning. It is also possible to create images in three dimensions, a process known as *single photon emission computerized tomography (SPECT)* when used in combination with gamma-emitting radionuclides, such as ^{99m}Tc, and positron emission tomography (PET) when used in combination with positron-emitting radionuclides, such as ^{18}F.

It is important to note that for the safe production of radiopharmaceuticals, the radiopharmacy must be designed to comply with, and procedures must follow, good manufacturing practice and good radiation protection practice. Radiopharmacists working in this field are part of a multidisciplinary team which includes physicians, physicists, radiochemists and technicians from the field of pharmacy, as well as nuclear medicine. As part of this team, they not only ensure that the radiopharmaceuticals will give high-quality clinical information, but also that they are safe for both patient and user alike.

Radionuclides used in nuclear medicine

Alpha-emitters

Alpha-decay is the process whereby a nucleus emits a helium nucleus, or alpha-particle. This commonly occurs with heavy nuclei (e.g. ^{226}Ra:$^{226}_{88}$Ra$\rightarrow^{222}_{86}$Rn+alpha).

Because they are heavy and positively charged, alpha-particles travel only short distances in air (~5 mm) and only micrometre distances in tissues. Their ionizing nature would result in a highly localized radiation dose if taken internally, and hence they tend not to be used as diagnostic radiopharmaceuticals, but may have a place as therapeutic agents.

Some alpha-emitters (e.g. ^{137}Cs), when encapsulated, are used as sealed sources, emitting X-rays or gamma-rays for radiotherapy applications. Here, the body is exposed to radiation externally in an attempt to treat malignant tumours.

Beta-emitters

Beta-decay occurs in two ways, one that involves the emission of a negatively charged beta$^-$-particle, or electron, and the other that involves the emission of a positively charged beta$^+$-particle, or positron.

Beta$^-$-emitters

Radionuclides which decay by beta$^-$-decay tend to have nuclei that are neutron rich. They attempt to reach a more stable state by the transformation of a neutron into a proton with the emission of a beta$^-$-particle (e.g. ^{32}P: $^{32}_{15}$P $\rightarrow$ $^{32}_{16}$S + beta$^-$). Despite beta$^-$-particles having a range in air of up to several metres, their range in tissues is only a few millimetres. Because of this and because of their highly ionizing nature, beta$^-$-emitters tend to be used in therapeutic radiopharmaceuticals (Table 16.1).

The principle of therapeutic treatment with radionuclides is to target the radionuclide to a specific tissue within the body, in an attempt to selectively damage or destroy that tissue. Ideally, therapeutic beta$^-$-emitting radionuclides should have energies of 0.5–1.5 MeV and a half-life of several days to provide a prolonged radiobiological effect.

The most widely used example of this is ^{131}I- sodium iodide, which is used in the treatment of hyperactive thyroid disease, and in certain thyroid tumours. Here, the physiological property of thyroid tissue is exploited to target the radionuclide to the site of action. Since thyroid tissue avidly takes up iodine in the normal synthesis of the hormone levothyroxine, radioactive iodine is also taken up and held in the thyroid tissue. Hence the radiation damage is targeted to the thyroid tissue specifically and the normal excretion of any excess iodine results in no significant damage to other organs and tissues.

Beta$^+$-emitters (positrons)

Radionuclides that emit positrons are becoming more widely used in nuclear medicine. In this transformation, a proton-rich nuclide attempts to achieve stability by converting a proton to a neutron with the emission of a positron (e.g. ^{11}C:$^{11}_6$C $\rightarrow$ $^{11}_5$S + beta$^+$ + gamma). The positron is very short-lived, since it interacts with an electron resulting in an annihilation reaction and the conversion of both particles into electromagnetic (EM) radiation. This EM radiation is in the form of two gamma-rays, each having energy of 0.511 MeV, which are emitted at an angle of 180° to each other.

When used in conjunction with a specialized gamma-camera, with detectors placed 180° apart, it

Table 16.1 Examples of radionuclides used in nuclear medicine

Mode of decay	Radionuclide	Radiopharmaceutical	Half-life	Clinical use
Beta$^-$-emitters	^{131}I	Sodium iodide capsules	8 days	Thyrotoxicosis, thyroid carcinomas
	^{89}Sr	Strontium chloride injection	50 days	Palliation of pain from bone metastases
Beta$^+$-emitters	^{15}O	^{15}O$_2$ gas	2.04 min	Brain blood flow imaging
	^{11}C	^{11}C-methionine	20.4 min	Prostate cancer
	^{13}N	^{13}N ammonia	9.97 min	Cardiac perfusion
	^{18}F	Fluorodeoxy-glucose injection	109.8 min	Tumour detection
Electron capture	^{111}In	Indium chloride solution	67 h	Antibody labelling
	^{123}I	Sodium iodide injection	13 h	Thyroid imaging
Isomeric transition	^{99m}Tc	Sodium pertechnetate injection	6 h	See Table 16.2
	^{81m}Kr	Krypton gas	13 s	Lung ventilation imaging

is possible to create images in all three dimensions, with the position of the radiopharmaceutical being very precisely known. This type of imaging technique is known as *positron emission tomography (PET)*. There are a number of positron emitting radionuclides which are becoming important tools in diagnostic imaging. Currently ^{18}F-labelled glucose, known as *^{18}F-fluoro deoxy-glucose* (^{18}F-FDG), is the most commonly used PET radiopharmaceutical in hospital practice and as a result the production processes for it will be described in simplified form and used as an example (see later). However, it should be noted there are four main positron emitters used to prepare radiopharmaceuticals (see Table 16.1). PET imaging with ^{18}F-FDG, in combination with X-ray computerized tomography (CT) is rapidly becoming an important imaging technique in the diagnosis of cancer.

Electron capture

Nuclei that are proton rich may, as an alternative to positron emission, capture electrons from the atom's electron orbital. This process results in the transformation of a proton to a neutron within the nucleus. The subsequent rearrangement of the electrons orbiting the nucleus results in a characteristic emission of X-rays or gamma-rays (e.g. ^{123}I:$^{123}_{53}I$ + electron→$^{123}_{53}Te$+gamma).

Radionuclides which decay by electron capture are useful in diagnostic imaging, since they emit gamma-rays; examples are given in Table 16.1.

Isomeric transition

Some radionuclides exist for measurable periods in excited, or isomeric, states prior to reaching ground state. This form of decay involves the emission of a gamma-ray and is known as *isomeric transition*. When radionuclides exist in this transitional state, they are known as *metastable*, which is denoted by the letter 'm' and written thus: ^{99m}Tc.

A simplified decay scheme for ^{99m}Tc-technetium is shown in Figure 16.1 where ^{99m}Tc's parent radionuclide, molybdenum (^{99}Mo), decays by beta$^-$-emission to the ground state ^{99}Tc either directly or indirectly.

The indirect route, which is the most common, involves the isomer ^{99m}Tc, which in turn decays from its metastable state to ^{99}Tc by isomeric transition.

Radionuclides which decay by this process are used in diagnostic imaging since they emit gamma-rays (see Table 16.1). It should be noted that ^{99m}Tc is the most widely used radionuclide in hospital radiopharmacy today, making up the radionuclide component of around 90% of the radiopharmaceuticals produced.

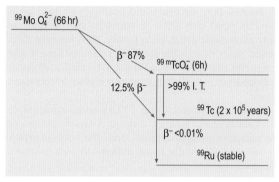

Fig. 16.1 Diagrammatic representation of ^{99}Mo decay.

For these reasons, the production processes for ^{99m}Tc-radiopharmaceuticals will be especially emphasized (see below).

Principles of ^{99m}Tc-radiopharmaceutical production

The physical and chemical properties of ^{99m}Tc make it nearly ideal for imaging purposes as outlined below:
- It has a 6-h half-life ($T_{1/2}$); long enough to allow imaging to take place in the working day, while also being short enough that patients are not radioactive for long periods (in 24 h, or 4 half-lives, the radioactivity will have decayed by 94%)
- ^{99m}Tc emits gamma-rays of 140 keV energy: ideal for use with the modern gamma-camera
- There are no particulate emissions that, if present, would add to the patient's radiation dose
- By purchasing a device known as a *$^{99}Mo/^{99m}Tc$ -generator*, ^{99m}Tc can be made readily available to the hospital site in a sterile and pyrogen-free form
- ^{99m}Tc has versatile coordination chemistry and will allow a large number of ligands to complex with it. By using different ligands in the radiopharmaceutical's formulation, a wide range of radiopharmaceuticals can be prepared in the radiopharmacy, providing for the many different investigations carried out in nuclear medicine departments (Table 16.2).

The production of ^{99m}Tc – the molybdenum/technetium generator

Radionuclides with long half-lives (e.g. ^{131}I, $T_{1/2}$=8 days) can be easily transported from production site to the user hospital. With shorter half-life radionuclides, e.g. ^{99m}Tc,

Table 16.2 Examples of ^{99m}Tc-radiopharmaceuticals

Radiopharmaceutical	Organ or tissue of distribution	Main clinical application
^{99m}Tc-sodium pertechnetate	Thyroid	Imaging the thyroid gland and ectopic tissue
	Salivary gland	Dynamic images of accumulation and drainage to show gland function
	Gastric mucosa	Presence of Meckel's diverticulum containing gastric mucosa
^{99m}Tc-methylene diphosphonate (MDP)	Skeleton	Bone metastases from carcinoma of lung, breast and prostate
^{99m}Tc-macro-aggregates of albumin (MAA)	Lung blood flow	Lung perfusion studies, most commonly for the diagnosis of pulmonary embolism
^{99m}Tc-exametazime (HMPAO)	Brain blood flow	Regional cerebral imaging in stroke and tumours
		Diagnosis of Alzheimer's dementia
^{99m}Tc-exametazime (HMPAO) labelled leucocytes	Infection or inflammation	Identification of abscesses associated with pyrexia of unknown origin. Extent of inflammatory bowel disease
^{99m}Tc-tetrofosmin	Heart	Cardiac perfusion imaging
^{99m}Tc-sestamibi (MIBI)	Heart	Cardiac perfusion imaging
^{99m}Tc-tin colloid	Liver	Location of hepatic tumours, abscesses and cysts. Detection of cirrhosis
^{99m}Tc-mercapto triglycine (MAG 3)	Kidney	Dynamic studies to study kidney function
^{99m}Tc-dimercapto-succinic acid (DMSA)	Kidney	Static imaging showing the kidney structure

this supply system would be extremely difficult. As a result, a device known as the *radionuclide generator* is used to provide ^{99m}Tc to the hospital site.

Radionuclide generators work on the principle that they contain a relatively long-lived 'parent' radionuclide that decays to produce a 'daughter' radionuclide. The chemical nature of parent and daughter are different, allowing separation of the daughter from the parent.

The molybdenum/technetium generator consists of ^{99}Mo (long-lived 'parent') absorbed onto an alumina-filled column, the ^{99}Mo being present in the form of molybdate (^{99}MoO$_4$$^{2-}$). ^{99}Mo decays to its 'daughter' radionuclide ^{99m}Tc, as pertechnetate, ^{99m}TcO$_4$$^-$ (see Fig. 16.1). The amount of ^{99m}TcO$_4$$^-$ grows as a result of the decay of ^{99}Mo, until a transient equilibrium is reached. At this point, the amount of ^{99m}Tc in the column appears to decay with the half-life of ^{99}Mo (Fig. 16.2).

By drawing a solution of sodium chloride 0.9% weight in volume (w/v) through the column, ^{99m}Tc is removed from the column in the form of sodium pertechnetate, Na^{99m}TcO$_4$. This process is known as *eluting the generator* and the resulting solution as the *eluate*. This process results in the production of a sterile solution of sodium pertechnetate that may now be used to make ^{99m}Tc-radiopharmaceuticals.

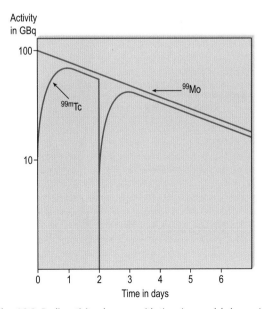

Fig. 16.2 Radioactivity changes with time in a molybdenum/technetium generator column.

^{99}Mo remains on the column where it decays to produce further ^{99m}Tc, the equilibrium being re-established about 23 h after elution. Elution of the generator is repeated daily to provide the radiopharmacy with a supply of ^{99m}Tc for 7–14 days, beyond which the yield of ^{99m}Tc becomes too small to be useful. Hospital radiopharmacies tend to buy generators on a weekly basis to provide a continuous supply of ^{99m}Tc.

Design of a ^{99m}Tc-generator

The design of a typical generator will be described by reference to the GE Healthcare generator, Drytec (Fig. 16.3). The main components of this generator are:

- A needle connected to the top end of the alumina column by tubing (it is this needle upon which a vial of IV Sodium Chloride Intravenous Infusion BP 0.9% w/v will be placed)
- A sterile alumina column to which is bound ^{99}Mo
- An elution needle which is connected to the bottom end of the alumina column
- Two 0.22-µm filters.

These components are housed within a compact plastic casing. The alumina column is encased in lead to give protection from the radiation.

Operating the generator is fairly straightforward. A vial of Sodium Chloride Intravenous Infusion BP 0.9% w/v, supplied with the generator, is first placed on the left-hand

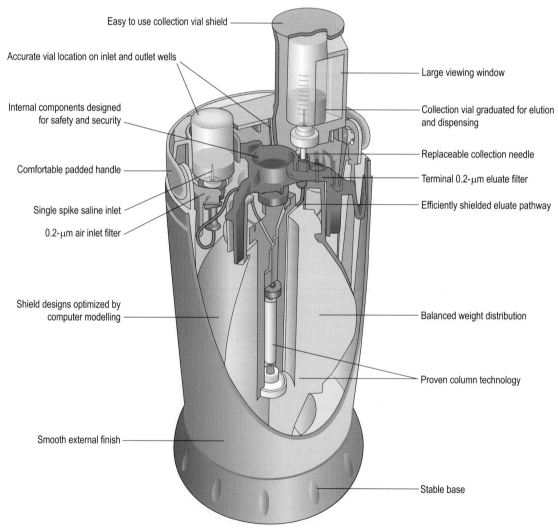

Easy to use collection vial shield

Accurate vial location on inlet and outlet wells

Internal components designed for safety and security

Comfortable padded handle

Single spike saline inlet

0.2-µm air inlet filter

Shield designs optimized by computer modelling

Smooth external finish

Large viewing window

Collection vial graduated for elution and dispensing

Replaceable collection needle

Terminal 0.2-µm eluate filter

Efficiently shielded eluate pathway

Balanced weight distribution

Proven column technology

Stable base

Fig. 16.3 The Drytec^{99m}Tc-generator. (Courtesy of GE Healthcare plc.)

needle (see Fig. 16.3). A sterile evacuated vial, also supplied with the generator, is placed in a lead pot designed for the elution process. Then by placing this on the elution needle, the vacuum draws sterile Sodium Chloride Intravenous Infusion BP 0.9% w/v from the vial through the column, and into the evacuated vial. When eluate has been collected, air enters the elution vial after first passing through the column. This dries the column as well as removing excess vacuum in the elution vial. The elution process is now complete and the vial may be removed from the generator.

The sterility of the eluates is maintained throughout the useful life of the generator by the following means:

- The eluting solution is terminally sterilized Sodium Chloride Intravenous Infusion BP 0.9% w/v
- Air entering the system passes through a 0.22-µm filter
- A terminal eluate 0.22-µm filter is placed between the column and the elution needle
- Between elutions, the needle is protected by a single-use, disposable, sterile needle guard.

The elution of the generator should be carried out in a Grade A environment (see Ch. 11).

Preparation of ^{99m}Tc-radiopharmaceuticals

The daily supply of ^{99m}Tc is provided by the elution of the generator, resulting in a sterile solution of sodium pertechnetate that is subdivided to provide the radioactive component of the radiopharmaceutical. Some nuclear medicine investigations use sodium pertechnetate alone as the radiopharmaceutical (see Table 16.2). In this case, preparation of sodium pertechnetate injection requires only the subdivision from the generator eluate, with perhaps some further dilution with Sodium Chloride Intravenous Infusion BP 0.9% w/v.

Other investigations, and these are in the majority, use radiopharmaceuticals that involve the chemical transformation of the sodium pertechnetate into another radiochemical form.

In order to make the preparation of ^{99m}Tc-radiopharmaceuticals as simple as possible, commercially available 'kits' are used to manufacture these radiopharmaceuticals. These kits allow the radiopharmacist, in the hospital environment, to transform the pertechnetate, via complex chemical reactions performed within the vial, into the desired radiopharmaceutical. This is achieved by the simple addition of pertechnetate into the vial followed by shaking to dissolve the contents.

A kit consists of a pre-packed set of sterile ingredients designed for the preparation of a specific radiopharmaceutical. Most commonly, the ingredients are freeze dried, enclosed within a rubber-capped nitrogen-filled vial. Normally, the kit contains sufficient materials to prepare a

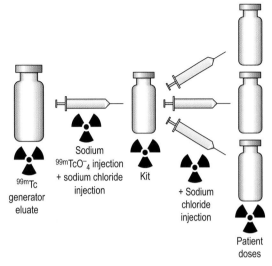

Fig. 16.4 Schematic representation of the preparation of patient doses of radiopharmaceuticals.

number of patient doses. In a typical formulation, the following may be found:

- The compound to be complexed to the ^{99m}Tc. These are known as *ligands* (e.g. methylene diphosphonate)
- Stannous ions (e.g. stannous chloride or fluoride) which are present as a reducing agent. The reduction of ^{99m}TcO$_4^-$ to a lower valance state is required to allow the ligands to form a complex with the ^{99m}Tc
- Other compounds that act as stabilizers, buffers or antioxidants.

An example of how ^{99m}Tc-radiopharmaceutical production may be performed is given below. The compounding procedures must be carried out within the facilities described in Chapter 11 using aseptic technique and carried out as 'closed' procedures (good manufacturing practice [GMP]).

The production method (Fig. 16.4) involves two simple steps:

Step 1. The freeze-dried kit is reconstituted by aseptically transferring the necessary activity of sodium pertechnetate using a sterile syringe and needle. This step may also include a further dilution of the eluate with a suitable diluent. The amount of activity withdrawn for the reconstitution of the kit vial depends on two factors:

- The number of patient doses to be manufactured
- The amount of activity required at injection time for each of the patient doses. The calculation would take into account the decay of ^{99m}Tc.

Manufacturers normally specify a maximum activity that may be added to the vial.

Step 2. The reconstituted kit is aseptically subdivided to provide each patient dose with sufficient activity to allow proper imaging after administration. As in Step 1, a diluent may be added to the final dose to give the desired radioactive concentration.

^{99m}Tc-radiopharmaceuticals must be administered on the day of production, for the following reasons:

- *Sterility.* Aseptically prepared pharmaceuticals should ideally be administered within a few hours of production, in accordance with GMP
- *Radioactivity.* ^{99m}Tc has a half-life of only 6 h
- *Radiochemical stability.* ^{99m}Tc-complexes are generally stable for a period between 4 and 8 h after production.

Principles of ^{18}F-fluoro deoxy-glucose (^{18}F-FDG) production

In the manufacture of ^{18}F-FDG, there are two main processes. First, there is the production of the radionuclide itself, which is produced in a cyclotron facility. This is followed by the radio-synthesis of the ^{18}F-FDG, which is carried out in an automated apparatus, known as a *synthesis module*. The resulting solution of ^{18}F-FDG has then to be sterilized and may have to be sub-dispensed in some way, so as to provide the injection in a ready to administer form. Since the ^{18}F-FDG has been synthesized, it will require analysis and other quality control checks prior to administration to the patient.

Radionuclide production

A cyclotron is a device used to produce radionuclides. It accelerates atomic or subatomic particles in a circular orbit, increasing the energy of the particles until a high-energy beam of particles is created. Once the particles have reached their maximum energy, they are extracted using high voltage and allowed to bombard target materials. The composition of the target material and the nuclear reactions that take place determine the radionuclides that are produced.

For ^{18}F production, the most common nuclear reaction used is the ^{18}O (p,n) ^{18}F reaction, where protons are produced from hydrogen gas and are accelerated until, at a required energy, a 'beam' of the protons are allowed to bombard a target of ^{18}O-enriched water ($H_2{}^{18}O$). ^{18}O is a naturally occurring isotope of oxygen, but much less abundant than the normal ^{16}O. By forcing a proton into the ^{18}O nucleus the now unstable nucleus ejects a neutron and the result is the production of ^{18}F – a positron-emitting radionuclide.

Radio-synthesis

2-[^{18}F] fluoro-2-deoxy-D glucose (^{18}F-FDG) may be prepared by various chemical pathways, but whatever radio-synthetic

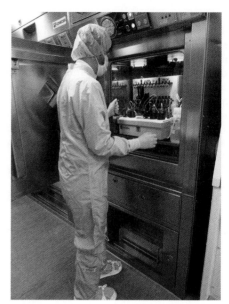

Fig. 16.5 Synthesis module for ^{18}F-FDG production (TRACER-labFx Synthesizer). Module located in lead-shielded (5.5 cm) specialized fume cupboard known as 'hot cell'. (Courtesy of GE Healthcare plc.)

route is used, it must be rapid to minimize the radiation risk and be of high yield. An automated apparatus, the synthesis module, is used to synthesize the ^{18}F-FDG to assure production efficiency and keep radiation exposure to a minimum. There are now commercially available synthesis modules such as the TRACERlabFx Synthesizer as shown in Figure 16.5, which are supplied with GMP standard raw materials and reagents for use in the module. Using this equipment, the following synthetic pathway is performed:

1. The ^{18}F-fluoride is adsorbed by an anion-exchange resin.
2. The retained ^{18}F-fluoride is eluted using an aqueous potassium carbonate solution.
3. A phase transfer catalyst (Kriptofix 222) dissolved in acetonitrile is then added, to bind the potassium ion and to enhance the nucleophilic reactivity of the ^{18}F-fluoride.
4. After evaporation of the solvents, the ^{18}F-fluoride is allowed to react with the reagent mannose triflate at elevated temperature (1,3,4,6-O-Acetyl-2-O-trifluoromethanesulfonyl-beta-D-mannopyranose). The structure of mannose triflate is similar to that of glucose with a leaving group (triflate) and four acetyl protecting groups to ensure the mannose ring undergoes nucleophilic substitution at the second carbon atom.
5. Hydrolysis under acidic or alkaline conditions also at elevated temperature yields 2-[^{18}F] fluoro-2-deoxy-D glucose (^{18}F-FDG).

Sterilization and sub-dispensing

Sterilization of the ^{18}F-FDG is achieved either by filtration through a 0.2-μm filter, although there are automated systems that use high temperature short sterilization cycles (e.g. 10 min cycle consisting of 4 min heat up; 135°C for 3.5 min; 2.5 min cool down). Sub-dispensing or fractionation of the bulk solution into patient doses is then carried out using robotic dispensing systems that perform the aseptic transfers, since the radiation hazard is too great for regular manual aseptic transfer. This aseptic manipulation is carried out within a specialized isolator specifically designed for handling PET radiopharmaceuticals.

Quality control

Since the ^{18}F-FDG has been synthesized, it must undergo stringent testing as outlined in the monograph given in the *European Pharmacopoeia*. A detailed description is beyond the scope of this chapter, but in summary the tests will include:

- Identification test
- Determination of pH
- Sterility test
- Determination of bacterial endotoxins
- Determination of chemical purity
- Determination of radionuclide purity
- Determination of radiochemical purity
- Determination of the radioactivity.

Facilities required for the production of radiopharmaceuticals

The majority of radiopharmaceuticals are intended for IV administration; therefore it is of paramount importance that these preparations are sterile. They also contain radionuclides with short half-lives that require their preparation and administration on the same day. Because of the thermal lability of some of these products, it is not possible to use terminal sterilization by autoclaving and hence these injections must be prepared using aseptic techniques. Here, highly skilled operators work with sterile ingredients within clean room facilities containing either laminar flow safety cabinets or isolators. The facilities for carrying out such manipulations are more fully described in Chapter 11, but there is specialized equipment as well as design criteria specifically for handling radiopharmaceuticals. More information can be found in Further Reading.

Radiation protection in the radiopharmacy

There are three basic principles to radiation protection:

- *Shielding.* By placing shielding around the radioactive source, the radiation dose rate may be reduced. Materials used as shielding must be appropriate to the type of radiation being emitted by the radionuclide. Plastic, Perspex, and metals of low molecular weight such as aluminium are appropriate materials for shielding beta-emitters. For gamma-emitters, high molecular weight metals such as lead and tungsten should be used. The thickness of shielding material necessary for gamma-emitters is dependent on the gamma-ray energy – the greater the energy, the thicker the shield required
- *Distance.* The radiation dose from a radioactive source is inversely proportional to the square of the distance (i.e. by doubling the distance the radiation dose is quartered)
- *Time.* Minimizing the time spent handling a radioactive source will reduce the radiation dose. It is important for new operators to practise the handling operation prior to working with radioactive materials.

In working practice, all three of these principles may be used in isolation or together, to reduce the radiation dose to the operator. For example, in the dispensing operation outlined in Figure 16.4, all vials containing radioactive material would be contained in a 3-mm lead pot. This will attenuate ^{99m}Tc's gamma-rays by a factor of approximately 1000. The syringes used to carry out the transfers would be only half full (i.e. 1 mL of radioactive solution would be transferred with a 2-mL syringe) in order to maximize the distance between the operator's fingers and the source, without compromising the accuracy of the dispensing operation.

The syringes, during the operation, should also be contained within a syringe shield. These are made of materials such as lead, tungsten, lead glass or lead acrylic, the latter two being transparent. Lead and tungsten syringe shields have lead glass/acrylic windows incorporated to allow the operator to see the graduations on the syringe. Alternatively, the whole syringe shield may be made of lead glass/acrylic which would have the advantage of giving greater visibility.

Handling the vials outside their lead pots should be carried out using long forceps and not with the fingers. The dispensing process should be carried out over a 'drip tray' that allows easy containment of any accidental spillage. It also should be carried out within a laminar flow safety cabinet or negative pressure isolator that provides operator protection as well as product protection (see Ch. 11).

The staff working in the radiopharmacy will be constantly monitored to assess their radiation exposure and to ensure compliance with safety legislation. Whole-body dose may be monitored with film badges and the radiation dose to the finger pulp with thermo-luminescent dosimeters.

Key points

- Radiopharmaceuticals may be used in therapy or diagnosis, the latter either as tracers or in imaging
- PET-CT imaging with ^{18}F-FDG is becoming an important imaging technique in the diagnosis of cancer
- ^{18}F-FDG may be prepared by first producing ^{18}F in a cyclotron, followed by the radio-synthesis of the ^{18}F-FDG, which is carried out in an automated apparatus, known as a *synthesis module*
- ^{99m}Tc is the most widely used radionuclide
- A molybdenum/technetium generator will provide a daily supply of ^{99m}Tc for 7–14 days, as sodium pertechnetate
- Reacting with a suitable ligand can chemically modify sodium pertechnetate. Different ligands give different bio-distributions, resulting in the wide range of scans that may be performed with ^{99m}Tc
- Radiation protection should be provided for operators using a combination of shielding, distance and time

Chapter | 17 |

Specialized services

Geoff Saunders

STUDY POINTS

- Pharmacy aseptic compounding services and the range of medicines prepared in them
- Equipment and procedures used in centralized cytotoxic reconstitution services
- Occupational health risks of cytotoxic drugs and the effective management of these risks
- Benefits of centralized, pharmacy-operated aseptic compounding services
- Scope and operation of a centralized intravenous additive service (CIVAS)

Introduction

This chapter describes the specialized services provided by hospital pharmacy departments in the provision of various aseptic dosage forms. These services may include: chemotherapy reconstitution services, centralized intravenous additive services (CIVAS), radiopharmacy services (see Ch. 16) and home-care services. In each case, the service involves the provision of aseptically-prepared medicines, which are often tailored to the specific needs of individual patients. This chapter introduces the scope, practice and pharmaceutical challenges of aseptic compounding services.

Cancer chemotherapy

The majority of chemotherapy doses are administered as injections or infusions. This offers the advantages of assured bioavailability, control over the rate and sequence of drug administration, and also the ability to stop administration immediately in the event of adverse effects. However, the parenteral route may be associated with complications such as infection, extravasation and thromboembolism. The majority of these drugs are given in the hospital setting.

Cytotoxic drugs are available as sealed vials containing freeze-dried powders or sterile, concentrated solutions, and are designed to provide an adequate shelf-life (usually >2 years). The freeze-dried powders require reconstitution with an appropriate diluent. Either may then require further dilution before being filled into syringes, infusion bags or infusion devices for administration.

Ambulatory infusion devices can be filled for use in the community by patients receiving home chemotherapy.

Occupational exposure risks

Cytotoxic drug exposure has been associated with various acute toxicities including headache, rash, nausea and dizziness. However, the more serious risks are related to the potential mutagenic, carcinogenic and teratogenic effects. Routes of exposure include ingestion, inhalation, needle-stick injury and skin contact – the most significant risk for occupational exposure.

In the UK, the requirements for safe handling of cytotoxic drugs are set out and enforced by the Health and Safety Executive. Pharmacy staff preparing cytotoxic agents must be fully trained in the necessary aseptic and safe handling techniques and must be fully aware of the potential health risks and the precautions that are required. Current opinion suggests that resources should be invested in appropriate equipment, staff training and competency assessment.

Published guidelines include the following areas of safe practice:

- Personnel training and competency
- Facilities and containment systems
- Techniques and precautions
- Dealing with spillage
- Disposal
- Labelling, packaging and distribution
  Useful guidelines on cytotoxic handling include *The Cytotoxics Handbook*.

Provision of a pharmacy-based chemotherapy preparation service

Protection of both the product and the staff involved in its preparation is technically demanding and requires carefully developed systems and procedures, together with extensive validation, which must be integrated with the principles of good pharmaceutical manufacturing practice (GMP). Capacity plans should ensure that the service is capable of meeting current and future demand; for example, the rising demand for targeted therapies.

Despite the challenges outlined above, it is important that pharmacy staff 'own' chemotherapy preparation services and take a clear lead. In the UK, from NPSA Alert 20 on injectable medicines, it is clear that application of the risk assessment guidelines places all cytotoxic drugs in the high-risk category. It is therefore essential that these medicines are prepared by specialized hospital pharmacy aseptic units or by appropriate commercial providers. Pharmacy staff offer a unique combination of skills and expertise, including the practice of aseptic technique, a wide clinical knowledge of cancer chemotherapy, familiarity with formulation and drug stability issues, the application of GMP, quality assurance (QA) and quality control (QC) to aseptic preparation and considerable experience in working with standard operating procedures (SOPs), batch documentation and checking procedures. These are key attributes that help to ensure the provision of safe, effective chemotherapy and contribute towards minimizing the risks of occupational exposure to drugs used in the treatment of cancer.

Training required for staff preparing cytotoxics

All personnel involved in preparing and handling cytotoxics require training and competency assessment in the appropriate techniques. On a practical level, all staff must be aware of the following, over and above standard aseptic technique and the application of GMP to aseptic preparation:

- Procedures required on receipt of a prescription for chemotherapy
- Completion of worksheets or batch documents

- Techniques for the safe handling and manipulation of cytotoxic drugs
- Safe storage and transportation of chemotherapy
- Background information on commonly used chemotherapy drugs and protocols
- Local and national policies and procedures.

Validation of operator techniques

Prior to commencing work on reconstitution of cytotoxics, an operator's competence in this field must be assessed.

- The operator is asked to carry out broth transfer simulations where solutions are transferred from one vial or container to another
- The broth-filled vials can then be incubated and examined for microbiological growth
- Operators must achieve negative results (no growth after incubation) on each occasion before they are deemed capable of preparing cytotoxic agents
- Typically, each operator and each process would be re-validated at least every 3 months and training procedures should be reviewed on a regular basis
- Operators routinely incorporate environmental monitoring tests such as settle plates and finger-dab plates into the production schedule as part of the QA process
- Expert guidance on the validation and monitoring of aseptic compounding has been published by the NHS
- Operator technique in the safe handling of cytotoxic drugs can be assessed by simulating aseptic transfer processes using a sterile solution containing a fluorescent dye, as splashes or spillage can be visualized using a portable ultraviolet lamp
- As with assessment of aseptic technique, safe handling should be evaluated using a combination of simulation and expert observation.

Documentation required for cytotoxics

On receipt of a prescription for a cytotoxic agent, a number of procedures must be undertaken. Figure 17.1 shows the areas of work in which a pharmacist may have involvement.

When the prescription is received, it is clinically checked by an experienced oncology pharmacist. The prescription must be validated against an approved chemotherapy protocol. It is essential that patients receive the correct number of cycles of treatment at the correct intervals. The British Oncology Pharmacy Association Standards for Prescription Verification for Systemic Anti Cancer Therapy provides detailed guidance.

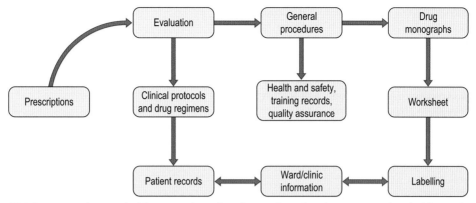

Fig. 17.1 Documentation required for cytotoxic services. (From Allwood et al. 2002, reproduced with permission.)

Information from the prescription is transferred to a worksheet or batch document and details of medicine(s) required, diluent and volume for reconstitution are recorded together with the number of drug vials required. Details of batch numbers and expiry date for each component used, all dose and dilution calculations, preparation methods, container(s) to be used, time and date of preparation and expiry of the final product are also required. Additionally, a sample label is attached to the worksheet. Most chemotherapy preparation units use pre-printed worksheets for each chemotherapy protocol, with a pharmacist-approved master document from which copies are made. Alternatively, some units use computer-based systems which contain a database of all approved chemotherapy protocols and produce batch documents and labels.

Labels should include the following information:
- Patient's name, hospital number and ward or clinic name
- Drug name, total quantity and final volume of infusion
- Vehicle in which the drug is prepared (e.g. 0.9% sodium chloride)
- Batch number, expiry date and storage conditions required
- Hospital pharmacy name and address
- Route of administration and infusion rate
- Inclusion of the term 'cytotoxic'.

When the worksheet is complete, the materials required are collected together and then subjected to an initial check before transfer to the designated clean room. After preparation has been completed, the finished product(s) and used or part-used vials are returned in the tray, together with batch documents, for labelling, inspection and release. Some cytotoxic agents require protection from light and are sealed in opaque plastic overwraps, which will also require labelling. The pharmacist responsible for the release of the prepared medicines will check all details on the worksheets and will reconcile the number of drug vials used in the preparation. If correct, the pharmacist will sign the worksheet or batch documents to signify approval, and the medicines are dispatched. All documents must be retained for up to 13 years after the date of preparation.

Cytotoxic preparation areas

In the UK, and in many parts of Europe, pharmaceutical isolators are used for cytotoxic preparation. In addition to providing aseptic conditions for preparation of the product, isolators are designed to protect the operator and the clean room environment from cytotoxic contamination. To achieve this, many isolators operate under negative pressure with respect to the clean room, and the exhaust air is externally ducted via a high-efficiency particulate air (HEPA) filter. All isolators should be located in a classified clean room.

It is generally accepted that isolators offer greater operator protection than open-fronted Class II safety cabinets. The main disadvantages of isolators include limited access for equipment and difficulties in cleaning and removing cytotoxic residues. Gas sterilizable isolators enable sterilization of the outer surface of vials and components used in the preparation process. Gases such as vaporized hydrogen peroxide are pumped into the isolator to sterilize the inside of the isolator and the outer surface of components in situ, prior to manipulation.

Techniques and precautions

When handling cytotoxics, it is vital that the appropriate protective clothing is worn. Operators using clean room facilities must wear appropriate clean room clothing, with the addition of chemotherapy gowns or armlets. These garments are non-shedding and have an absorbent surface and impermeable backing. Full clean room suits are worn beneath the chemotherapy gown, so it is important to ensure that the clean room temperature is carefully controlled. Gloves designed specifically for cytotoxic handling are available and these are normally fabricated from a nitrile material. Gloves should be worn for handling cytotoxic drug vials outside the clean rooms, as these can be contaminated with cytotoxic residues on the outer surface.

Product segregation is crucial in all aseptic work to avoid any risk of product mix up, and only one product or one batch of product is prepared at any one time.

Reconstitution procedures

When carrying out reconstitution procedures, certain precautions must be taken:
- Vials and outer packs of consumables should be sprayed with sterile 70% alcohol and wiped with a sterile swab before being introduced into the clean room, and the process repeated before introducing these materials into the isolator or Class II cabinet workstation. Rubber stoppers on vials should be swabbed with a sterile swab prior to removal of liquid
- Transfer of liquids to and from vials requires the insertion of a venting needle with hydrophobic filter into the vial, or the use of a vented reconstitution device. These devices ensure pressure equalization and reduce the risk of aerosol generation
- Luer lock syringes with wide-bore needles should be used for all procedures to allow free flow in the fluid pathway and to avoid the risk of syringes and needles becoming disconnected during fluid transfer
- To ensure that no further additions are made outside the pharmacy preparation area, all completed products in syringe form should be sealed with a blind hub before removal from the cytotoxic cabinet (Fig. 17.2). An additive plug or cap must be placed on each minibag once additions are complete.

The vials that contain cytotoxic agents are effectively a closed system, which contains either a powder requiring reconstitution or a drug concentrate requiring withdrawal from the vial into a syringe. In each case, equalization of pressure within the vial is required to allow withdrawal from it, and is achieved by inserting a sterile 0.2-mm hydrophobic filter venting needle into the vial to facilitate liquid transfer. Ordinary needles with no hydrophobic filter must not be used for venting due to the risk of leakage of cytotoxic solution from the needle. Alternatively, reconstitution devices are available to help with the reconstitution process. Some of these devices consist of a small plastic spike with an integral hydrophobic filter. These devices are useful for rapid transfer of solutions, but the large needle bore can produce large holes in the rubber bung of cytotoxic vials, thus increasing the risk of leakage. The CytoSafe needle is a commonly used example of this type of product. This device consists of a needle which is vented to allow equilibrium of

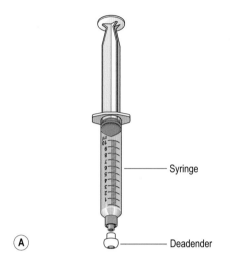

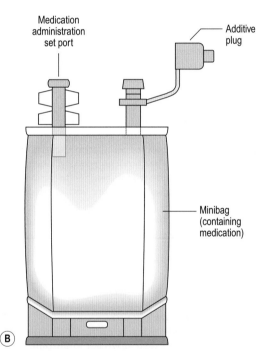

Fig. 17.2 (A) Syringe with deadender or blind hub in position. (B) Minibag with additive plug.

pressure between the vial and the syringe. It is useful for reconstitution of large vials or when more than one vial is required for a dose (Fig. 17.3). However, care must be taken when withdrawing or adding liquid to a vial as the filter may become blocked.

'Closed systems' using needle-free technologies have been designed for cytotoxic handling. These devices

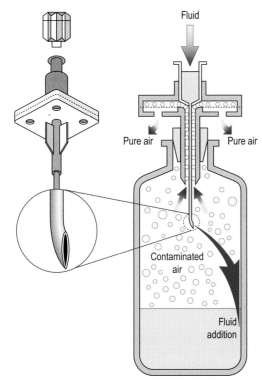

Fig. 17.3 (A) CytoSafe needle and (B) reconstitution set-up.

virtually eliminate the risks of cytotoxic aerosol formation and operator needle-stick injuries. An example of this type of device is the Tevadaptor (Fig. 17.4). This system comprises a vial adaptor to access the drug vial, and a syringe adaptor which fits securely onto a Luer lock syringe and enables needle-free docking with the vial adaptor. The closed reconstitution systems have been shown in studies to be effective in reducing cytotoxic contamination.

Dealing with cytotoxic spillage

In the event of a cytotoxic spillage, the problem should be dealt with immediately to prevent the spread of contamination. A written policy on dealing with spillages should be prepared. Most policies are based on a spillage kit which contains all the required materials to deal with a spill. Spillage kits should be available in pharmacy preparation units, in wards/clinics and in transport vehicles.

If the spillage has come in contact with the skin, the contaminated area should be washed thoroughly with soap and water. Contact with eyes should be dealt with by irrigation with a sodium chloride eyewash, and medical help sought. In the event of a needle-stick injury, the puncture wound should be encouraged to bleed and the area

should again be thoroughly washed. All incidents should be reported.

Disposal of cytotoxic waste

Cytotoxic waste materials are regarded as 'hazardous waste' and should be placed in a purple coloured plastic bag, sealed and labelled with a cytotoxic warning label ready for disposal by incineration. Sharp objects including needles, syringes, ampoules and vials should be placed in a sharps bin, which is made of rigid plastic and does not allow leakage of cytotoxic waste. When the sharps bin is full, it should be sealed with 'cytotoxic' warning tape and disposed of by incineration.

Packaging of cytotoxic infusions

Cytotoxic infusions should be packaged in a labelled, hermetically sealed overwrap. This has two functions: containment of any leak from the infusion and protection of staff from any cytotoxic residues. Ideally, the infusions should be transported in a rigid, closed plastic box to protect from any mechanical trauma.

Management of the chemotherapy workload

It is evident from the above text that chemotherapy preparation is very labour-intensive. There is a clear tendency to move from in-patient treatment of cancer patients on hospital wards to chemotherapy outpatient clinics. This can place significant workload pressures on pharmacy chemotherapy units, partly because several patients often arrive for treatment at the same time, and also because blood test results and other patient-specific data are required before the oncologist is able to confirm the chemotherapy dose and allow treatment to proceed.

Various strategies have been employed to manage these problems. In many centres, it is possible to organize patients' blood samples 2 days before the patient is due to visit the outpatient clinic for treatment. This enables prescriptions to be 'pre-written', so that pharmacy can prepare batch documents and tray-up consumables on the day before treatment.

Many oncology centres have adopted the approach of 'dose-banding'. Individual patient doses are calculated in the normal way, but the dose is then fitted to pre-defined dose ranges or 'bands'. These standard doses are provided from a limited range of standard pre-filled syringes or infusion bags, either singly or in combination. In practice, five or six standard pre-fills are needed to provide the required range of standard doses.

There is no doubt that managing chemotherapy services is a very challenging task. Operating a patient-focused

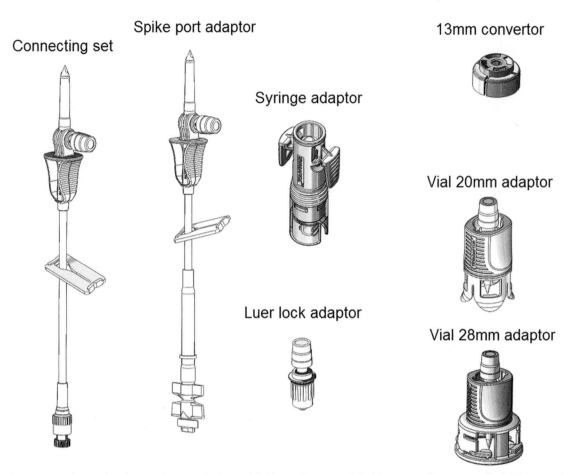

Connecting set

Spike port adaptor

Syringe adaptor

Luer lock adaptor

13mm convertor

Vial 20mm adaptor

Vial 28mm adaptor

Fig. 17.4 Tevadaptor closed cytotoxic reconstitution and fluid transfer system.

service that meets clinical needs within the confines of limited resources requires innovation, organization and regular communication with medical and nursing colleagues. The service should be carefully monitored and key outcomes, such as errors and patient waiting times, should be audited on a regular basis.

Centralized intravenous additive service (CIVAS)

The Breckenridge Report (1976) made recommendations that IV infusions should be prepared, where possible, by hospital pharmacies. The provision of an IV additive service did not commence until the 1980s and then only in a limited number of hospitals.

Currently, a large proportion of hospital pharmacists in the UK and many European countries provide a CIVAS, and this is augmented by a growing number of commercial compounding units. Despite these developments, it is estimated that of all infusions prepared in UK hospitals, less than 40% are prepared in pharmacy CIVAS units.

Scope of a CIVAS

A CIVAS is set up to provide a range of parenteral dosage forms suitable for administration to patients. A CIVAS can provide the following:

- IV antibiotics, antivirals, antifungals and steroids
- Patient-controlled analgesia, and other opioid infusions for postoperative analgesia and palliative care
- Epidural analgesics infusions
- Ambulatory infusion devices for various IV therapies at home
- Electrolyte infusions (that are not commercially available).

Given that CIVAS are resourced to provide only a proportion of the IV additive/compounding needs of a hospital, they normally prioritize the services offered according to clinical risk. Accordingly, CIVAS-produced infusions often include antibiotics for neonates and paediatric patients which require extensive dilution to the required doses. Economic factors can also influence which infusions are prepared in CIVAS units. Many IV medicines contain no preservative and are designed for single use only. However, subject to validated infusion stability, it is possible for a CIVAS unit to prepare a batch of infusions for several days' use, or even longer, so reducing or eliminating drug wastage.

Provision of a CIVAS

The main goals of providing a CIVAS should include:
- Improved patient safety
- Improved use of hospital resources
- Improved services to patients, particularly with home infusions
- Improved pharmacy control and reduced risk of medication errors.

Although there are compelling reasons for the provision of pharmacy CIVAS in all major hospitals, it is important in presenting a balanced argument to be aware of potential disadvantages to the hospital and healthcare system:
- Increased pharmacy expenditure, diverting funds from other healthcare services
- Pharmacy CIVAS, once established, should be available 24 hours a day, including weekends and public holidays
- There is a potential risk of de-skilling ward staff in the preparation of drug infusions
- Some wards and departments may be difficult to service, e.g. accident and emergency, because doses of some drugs may be required urgently
- The capacity of the CIVAS is not infinite, but there will always be pressures to add new drugs to the service as soon as these enter clinical use.

Many of these problems can be overcome through good communication, both within the pharmacy department and with medical and nursing staff. A service level agreement is a useful device for ensuring that all stakeholders know their responsibilities and that the service operates within the confines of the available resources.

Quality assurance

All procedures used during preparation of CIVAS doses must be fully validated and documented. Procedures must also be audited and be subject to in-process monitoring. Staff preparing IV products should complete appropriate batch documents and adhere to authorized SOPs and published guidelines. As with the chemotherapy preparation service described previously, there are various elements to be considered as part of the decision-making process for the release of CIVAS medicines for administration to patients. Clean room over-pressures should be recorded at least daily, and HEPA filter integrity checks should be carried out at least on an annual basis, or in the event of any deviation from defined operating conditions.

Records will be kept for all IV medicines prepared and will include the batch numbers of products used during reconstitution procedures. This ensures that in the event of a product recall or any problems with an IV medicine, a full audit trail documenting all aspects of the process can be reviewed.

Validation of procedures

Validation of processes and operator technique for CIVAS is almost identical to the validations necessary for chemotherapy preparation.

Infusion stability and shelf-life assignment

The assignment of a shelf-life or expiry date to any aseptically prepared medicine is a rigorous, evidence-based process, which requires expert interpretation of physical and chemical stability data and a clear understanding of the level of protection afforded to prevent microbiological contamination during the aseptic preparation process.

In the UK, aseptic medicines prepared requiring pharmacist supervision of the process are restricted to a maximum shelf-life of 7 days, and then only if there is evidence to support this. On the other hand, aseptic medicines made under a manufacturer's 'specials' licence issued by the MHRA can be assigned any reasonable shelf-life, providing this is supported by rigorous evidence.

Stability data for CIVAS infusions, including cytotoxic drugs, can be sourced from a number of reference books. In many cases, it will be necessary to search the scientific and professional literature for original stability study reports and, on some occasions, the drug manufacturer may be willing to share extended stability data. Whatever the source of information, stability data should always be subjected to critical appraisal before it is used in the assignment of infusion shelf-lives.

Assessment of infusion stability is a key responsibility of any pharmacist managing a CIVAS. In the case of infusions that are outsourced from commercial compounding units, it is essential that clear and robust evidence is available to support the assigned shelf-life. Care must be exercised when attempting to extrapolate published stability data to infusions with variations in the concentration, diluents, or container used. Expert review and a written justification are required to validate a shelf-life where there is any variation to the conditions under which the stability data were obtained.

Consideration must also be given to the transportation and storage of aseptically prepared medicines. Cold chain transport systems must be fully validated to ensure that the stability of infusions is not compromised, and the storage temperatures should be monitored at least daily, but preferably by continuous monitoring and data logging.

Key points

- Cancer chemotherapy can include treatment with cytotoxic drugs and biological 'targeted' therapies
- There are significant occupational exposure risks to healthcare workers who handle cytotoxic drugs
- Compliance with safe handling guidelines, combined with use of protective equipment, containment facilities and validated technique can minimize unplanned cytotoxic exposure
- Use of strict aseptic conditions minimizes the risk of microbiological contamination during preparation

- Detailed SOPs for preparation and administration of chemotherapy must be prepared and implemented
- All personnel involved in provision of a centralized cytotoxic reconstitutions service must be trained and validated in all relevant procedures and techniques
- Transfer of solutions between cytotoxic drug vials and syringes must be carried out using a hydrophobic venting pin or a purpose-designed transfer device, to avoid the generation of aerosols
- Drug stability is a key issue in assigning infusion shelf-lives, particularly those used for home infusion
- Increased use of chemotherapy outpatient or day-case clinics can place significant pressures on the workload of the pharmacy chemotherapy unit
- New strategies such as 'dose-banding' are useful to manage chemotherapy workload
- A CIVAS can provide a wide range of aseptically prepared medicines for hospital and domiciliary use
- Potential benefits of CIVAS include reduced risk of medication errors, improved use of resources, better services to patients and pharmacy control
- Most doses are provided from CIVAS as either pre-filled syringes or minibags

Chapter 18

Appliances

Ian Smith

STUDY POINTS

- What appliances do pharmacists dispense?
- What makes an ideal wound dressing?
- What can be supplied for dressing a wound?
- What appliances are available for urinary incontinence?
- The appliances available for a patient with a stoma
- How to supply graduated compression hosiery
- How to supply a truss

Introduction

In addition to dispensing medicines, pharmacists have traditionally had a role in dispensing and supplying appliances. Appliances are sometimes termed as *medical devices*. In the European Union, there is a requirement that all appliances have a CE marking on them. This indicates that the product conforms to the relevant medical device directives laid down by the EU. There are some medical devices which are exempt from the CE marking requirement, an example of which would be made-to-measure hosiery.

In the UK, only the appliances which are listed in the *Drug Tariff* can be supplied on an NHS prescription.

The main types of appliance which pharmacists supply are wound dressings and incontinence and stoma products. Pharmacists are also required to supply and to measure and fit hosiery and trusses. Other appliances which pharmacists can supply include needles and syringes, bandages, ear syringes and peak flow meters.

Wound dressings

When the skin becomes damaged, it will undergo a process of wound healing. The speed and mechanism of the healing of the wound will depend on the degree of tissue loss and the depth and site of the wound. One major concern is that the wound may become infected.

The wound healing process consists of four overlapping phases:

1. *Haemostasis.* This is not always considered a phase in all publications. Bleeding is stopped by a combination of vasoconstriction and coagulation. It happens immediately the wound has occurred and can last from a few seconds to a few days, depending on the wound.
2. *Inflammation.* This is cleansing and removal of debris. This phase starts a few hours after haemostasis and can last a few days. The inflammatory response leads to redness, heat and swelling. Macrophages and polymorphs in the blood begin to clean the wound of debris, damaged tissues and bacteria. This leads to the production of exudate and the wound can become macerated.
3. *Proliferation.* This is characterized by granulation and vascularization. This starts after a few days and continues for a few weeks. It is the stage when the wound is rebuilt.
4. *Maturation or epithelialization.* At this final stage of wound healing, the collagen is remodelled.

From the phases required for healing, it can be seen that for effective wound healing the wound needs an adequate blood supply and nutrients, particularly vitamin C.

Therefore some conditions which affect the flow of blood to the wound might affect the speed of the healing process, such as diabetes or vascular disease. Certain drugs can also affect the wound healing process, such as cytotoxics.

In the past, wound dressings were used mainly to protect the wound and keep the area clean and warm. A greater understanding of the wound healing process has led to more advanced dressings. Understanding the different types of dressings and the wounds they treat requires a degree of specialism.

An ideal wound dressing should:
- Provide a moist, warm environment
- Remove excess exudate
- Be oxygen permeable but not permeable to bacteria
- Protect the wound from further damage
- Be easily removed and not required to be changed too frequently
- Not cause harm through being toxic, causing an allergic response or leaving particles
- Be cost-effective with a good shelf-life.

Wound dressings can be categorized in the following ways.

Basic wound contact dressings

- *Low adhesive dressings*: these are tulle (open weave fabric with yellow or white soft paraffin, e.g. Paratulle) or knitted viscous primary dressing (e.g. N-A Dressing)
- *Absorbent dressings*: these are further categorized into those for lightly, moderate to heavy and heavy exudating wounds
- *Lightly exudating wound dressings* are absorbent perforated dressings with an adhesive border (e.g. Mepore) and absorbent perforated plastic film faced dressings (e.g. Melolin)
- *Moderate to heavy absorbent dressings* include absorbent cellulose dressings with a fluid repellent backing (e.g. Mesorb)
- *Heavy exudating wound dressings* include a number of polymer dressings, some of which also contain cellulose (e.g. DryMax Extra).

Advanced wound dressings

- *Hydrogel dressings*: these are used to give the wound moisture as they are a polymer matrix which contains 96% water
- *Vapour permeable film and membrane*: these are impermeable to fluids and bacteria but permeable to air and water vapour. They are available with or without an absorbent pad

- *Soft polymer dressings*: these are available with or without an absorbent pad or biocellulose
- *Hydrocolloid dressings*. A number of hydrocolloids are available, e.g. pectin and gelatin. These form a gel when exposed to the exudate, and promote moist wound healing. These dressings are combined with a semi-permeable film, and come with or without adhesive
- *Foam dressings*: these contain polyurethane foam which absorbs the exudate. They can be adhesive or non-adhesive, and can come with or without a plastic film backing. They are categorized further in the BNF into those for lightly, lightly to moderate and moderate to heavy exudating wounds
- *Alginate dressings*: these are made from the alginic acid derived from brown seaweed. These dressings are highly absorbent, which makes them useful in exuding wounds. They are available as dressings or sheets and can be adhesive or non-adhesive
- *Capillary action dressing*. Hydrophilic fibres in the dressing draw up the exudate. Low-adhesive wound contact layers on either side of the fibres prevent any the fibres contaminating the wound
- *Odour absorbent dressings*: these dressings contain activated charcoal to reduce the odour coming from the wound
- *Antimicrobial dressings*: these dressings contain honey, silver, iodine or other antimicrobials to lower the number of bacteria in an infected wound.

Urinary incontinence

There are two main types of urinary incontinence:
1. Stress incontinence is caused by an action which raises intra-abdominal pressure such as sneezing, coughing or laughing.
2. Urge incontinence, of which enuresis is one type, is when the patient gets the urge to urinate but does not reach the toilet in time.

Stress and urge incontinence account for 90% of cases. Urinary incontinence is more common in females than males and the incidence increases in both sexes with age.

There are a number of appliances available for the management of urinary incontinence in men and women. In the UK, some of these devices are available on the NHS and these are listed in the *Drug Tariff*. Incontinence pads and garments are not available on the NHS in the UK.

Urinary catheters

These are tubes which are passed into the bladder to allow the drainage of urine from the bladder.

The main types of urinary catheters are Nélaton and Foley. Nélaton catheters are long tubes. Foley catheters have a balloon that is inflated by filling it with a liquid, normally sterile water. This balloon acts as a self-retaining device and holds the catheter in place in the bladder. The balloons come in different sizes, which are expressed in millilitres: 3-mL and 5-mL balloons are used in children and 10-mL and 30-mL in adults.

Catheters come in different lengths and diameters and are also made from different materials.

Materials

The material the catheter is made from will affect how long it can remain in place. Latex is suitable only short term. The latex can be coated with Teflon or silicone and this will increase the time it can be left in the bladder and not removed. Catheters made of silicone can be kept in place the longest.

Diameter

The Charrière (Ch) system is used to describe the different diameters. Only even numbers are used in this system and the bigger the number the larger the external diameter of the tube, ranging from 6 Ch (2 mm) to 30 Ch (10 mm). Sizes between 14 Ch and 18 Ch are the most common diameters used in adults. Paediatric catheters are usually between 6 Ch and 10 Ch.

Length

Differences in anatomy will mean that males require longer tubes than females. In males, the tubes are about 40 cm long and in females about 20 cm, hence the catheters are described as male, female or paediatric.

In males, an alternative to using a catheter is to use a latex sheath which fits over the penis. Some sheaths require another device to keep them in place.

Catheters or sheaths can then be connected to a drainage bag which will collect the urine. The volume of urine the bag holds varies. Some are intended to be worn on the leg so the patient can be mobile and some are intended for use when the patient is in bed. The drainage bag can be emptied of urine via a tap at times convenient to the patient or carer.

Stoma

Stomas or ostomies can be made surgically from the bowel, either the colon (colostomy) or ileum (ileostomy) or can be made from the ureters (urostomy – a piece of bowel is also used) or ureterostomy. An opening on the surface of the body is made through which the bowel or ureters drain the waste materials from the body. The stoma can be either permanent or temporary.

The colostomy is the most common type of stoma for which a pharmacist will supply appliances.

Colostomy and ileostomy appliances

The main type of appliance a pharmacist or appliance contractor supplies is used to collect the waste material which is being discharged from the stoma. The stoma, unlike the rectum, does not have sphincter muscles so the drainage of waste cannot be controlled. The appliance consists of a bag for collection, with some system for attaching the bag to the body. In addition to these collection devices, stoma caps, bag covers, deodorants and skin protectors are available.

Stoma bags

For a collection system to be effective it should have the following features:
- Comfortable to wear
- Does not leak and protects the skin from irritation
- Does not smell
- Not visible or noticeable (does not emit a noise)
- Easy to empty and change
- Able to hold the required amount of waste.

Stomas vary in size. This means that it is important to get a bag with the right diameter hole to fit the stoma and to prevent leaking and damage to the surrounding skin. The size of the stoma may change with time so it is important that patients be re-assessed.

The bags used for stomas can be drainable or non-drainable. The choice of appliance will depend on the nature of the waste being discharged. This can range from liquid to solid depending where along the bowel the stoma is, i.e. the nearer the stoma is to the rectum, the more solid will be the discharge.

If the appliance consists of the bag and is the means of attaching it to the body, it is called a *one-piece appliance*. If the method of attaching the bag to the body is separate from the bag, it is a *two-piece appliance*. With a two-piece system, you do not need to change the attachment on the body every time you change the bag.

The appliance can be adhesive so it sticks to the body or non-adhesive, which normally means it is held in place by a belt.

Some bags come with filters which are useful to prevent the bag from expanding if the patient is passing flatus.

Stoma caps or plugs can be used instead of a bag when the patient is able to predict when the bowel movement will happen. They may also be useful for short-term use when a patient is doing exercise or swimming.

Bag covers are used to cover the bag to make it less visible or to make the bag more comfortable to wear.

Unless the skin around the stoma is smooth and flat and the appliance fits precisely, it is possible that the waste from the stoma will come into contact with the skin. This can then lead to irritation and pain. Skin fillers and protectors are available to prevent this from happening.

Graduated compression hosiery

Graduated compression hosiery available on the NHS comes in three classes which are based on the degree (amount of pressure) of compression they give at the ankle, measured in millimetres of mercury (mmHg). They are mainly indicated for varicose veins but can also be used in the treatment and prevention of leg ulcers and oedema. The three classes are:

- Class 1 – light support (14–17 mmHg)
- Class 2 – medium support (18–24 mmHg)
- Class 3 – strong support (25–30 mmHg).

Hosiery comes in different lengths (thigh length or below knee), different knits (circular, flat bed, net), different sizes (e.g. small, medium and large) and different colours.

One of the roles of a pharmacist is to ensure that the hosiery is the right size for the patient and that they know how to put it on. The NHS pays an additional professional fee for the measuring and fitting of hosiery.

Sometimes a patient may not be a standard or stock size and, in this situation, the pharmacist will be required to measure the patient and will then order a made to measure stocking from the manufacturer.

There are also a number of accessories available for supply with hosiery to either help in putting them on or keeping them in place when they are on.

Trusses

Trusses are appliances used for abdominal hernias. A hernia occurs when an organ of the body protrudes through a cavity that is normally meant to keep it contained. If the abdominal muscle weakens, there is a chance that a hernia or rupture can occur. This is where the bowel protrudes through the abdominal wall. This is usually due to the fact that the abdominal wall has a number of weak points and with age, these weaken further. Hernias can also arise from an event which increases the pressure on the abdomen, such as coughing, lifting or straining on defecation. Hernias can be repaired by surgery. If a patient cannot undergo surgery or is waiting to have surgery, a truss can be fitted.

The purpose of the truss is to plug the hole in the abdominal wall and therefore prevent the bowel from coming through it. This helps prevent the hernia from becoming larger and reduces the chance the hernia will become strangulated. Strangulation is when the blood flow is restricted, due to the fact the bowel is trapped by the abdominal wall and can lead to complications where the bowel swells and may burst and peritonitis could ensue.

Other types of hernia

There are a number of hernias for which trusses are available:

- *Umbilical hernia*: happening around the umbilicus. Very rare and can be fitted with an elastic band umbilical truss
- *Femoral hernia*: more common in women and happens where the femoral blood vessel leaves the abdomen at the top of the leg. A spring truss with a femoral pad can be fitted to this hernia
- *Incisional hernia*: happens where the abdomen has been cut during surgery.

Inguinal and scrotal hernias

The commonest abdominal hernia happens at the point where the inguinal canal, which in men carries the spermal cord (vas deferens) to the testes, leaves the abdomen. This is called an 'inguinal hernia'. The bowel can follow the canal downward and can end up in the scrotal sac. If the lump caused by the bowel is below the pubic arch, the hernia is called a 'scrotal hernia'.

When a pharmacist receives a prescription for a truss, it should contain the following information:

- The position of the hernia – inguinal, scrotal, and which side it is on
- The type of belt – elastic band or spring
- The number of pads – single or double. The patient may have a hernia on both sides of the abdomen
- The type of pad used – inguinal or scrotal.

It is part of the service agreement with the NHS that pharmacists measure and fit trusses and an endorsement on a prescription of 'measured and fitted' attracts an additional professional fee.

Hiatus hernia

This is common and is a result of the stomach going into the chest cavity through the hiatus, which is the point where the oesophagus goes through the diaphragm. As this is internal, it would not warrant treatment with a truss.

Key points

- Pharmacists are required to supply appliances as well as medicines
- There are four stages involved in wound healing
- There are large numbers of wound dressings available to dress different types of wound
- Catheters vary in material, length and diameter
- There are different types of stoma
- Graduated compression hosiery comes in three classes
- Pharmacists may be required to measure and fit hosiery and trusses

Chapter 19

Routes of administration and dosage forms

Arthur J. Winfield

Introduction

Following the administration of a medicine, the drug has to reach its site of action or receptor in order to produce an effect. How this is achieved is often a complex process affected by many factors. The first stage will be the release of the drug from the dosage form, to be followed by absorption into the body (unless it is for a surface effect at the site of administration). There is then a distribution process, usually in the blood, which will take the drug to the site of action. As soon as it is in the body, metabolic processes, especially in the liver, will start to change the drug, and the elimination process will also commence. A detailed discussion of these processes is outside the scope of this book, although it does have a significant impact on the choice of both the route of administration and the actual dosage form. There is a growing awareness that the correct choices can have an important impact on therapeutic outcomes for the patient. This chapter will review the various routes of administration used for drug delivery and discuss some of their advantages and disadvantages. Brief details of a variety of dosage forms are also given. Figure 19.1 illustrates the principal routes of administration.

Routes of administration

The oral route

The oral route can produce either a systemic or a local effect. For a systemic effect, the drug, formulated in either a solid or a liquid form, is absorbed from the gastrointestinal tract (GIT). This is the most commonly used route for drug administration. There are several reasons for this:

- From a patient's point of view, it is the simplest route
- Self-administration of drugs can be carried out
- If used properly, it is also the safest route.

However, there are disadvantages which should be borne in mind:

- The onset of action is relatively slow
- Absorption from the GIT may be irregular
- Some drugs are destroyed by enzymes and other secretions found in the GIT
- As the blood supply from the GIT passes through the liver via the hepatic portal system, it is subject to hepatic metabolism before it enters the systemic circulation. This is called *first pass* or *pre-systemic metabolism*
- Drug solubility may be altered by the presence of other substances in the GIT, e.g. calcium
- Gastric emptying is very variable and can be influenced by factors such as food, drugs, disease state and posture. Not only does it affect the onset of action, but if it is extended it may cause a drug to be inactivated by gastric juices owing to prolonged contact

1 Buccal (inside mouth)
2 Oral (swallow)
3 Sublingual (under tongue)
4 Nasal
5 Rectal
6 Vaginal
7 Inhalation (to lungs)
8 Eye
9 Ear

10 Parenteral
  a Intravenous
  b Subcutaneous
  c Intramuscular
  d Intraspinal
Topical – skin (any site)

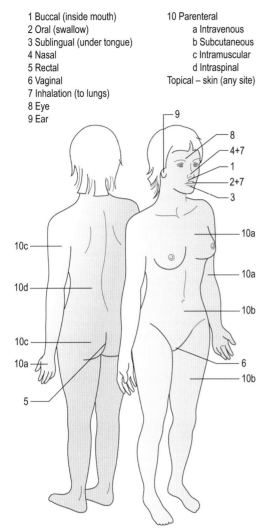

Fig. 19.1 Diagrammatic representation of the main routes of administration.

- It is an unsuitable route of administration in unconscious or vomiting patients and for immediate pre- or postoperative use.

The buccal routes

A drug is administered by these routes by being formulated as a tablet or spray and is absorbed from the buccal cavity. The highly vascular nature of the tongue and buccal cavity, and the presence of saliva, which can facilitate the dissolution of the drug, make this a highly effective and useful route for drug administration. It can also be used for a local action.

Two sites are used for absorption from the buccal cavity:

- For sublingual absorption, the area under the tongue is used. This gives a very fast onset of action of the drug, but duration of action is usually short
- For buccal absorption, the buccal sulcus is used. This is the area between the upper lip and the gum. Tablets formulated for absorption from the buccal sulcus give a quick onset of action, but will also give a longer duration of action than the sublingual route. This route can also administer drugs with a longer half-life, for an extended duration of action.

It is important that patients are made aware of the difference between the two sites and they should be given full instructions on how to administer their tablets, to ensure maximum benefit. (For details of suitable patient instructions, see Ch. 3.)

The advantages of the buccal route:

- There is a relatively quick onset of action
- Drugs are absorbed into the systemic circulation, thereby avoiding the 'first pass' effect
- Drugs can be administered to unconscious patients
- Because the tablet is not swallowed, antiemetic drugs can be given by this route.

The rectal route

For administration by this route, drugs are formulated as liquids, solid dosage forms and semi-solids (see Ch. 9). The chosen preparation is inserted into the rectum from where the drug is released to give a local effect, or it may be absorbed to give a systemic effect.

The rectum is supplied by three veins, namely the middle and inferior (lower) rectal veins, which drain directly into the systemic circulation and the upper rectal vein, which drains into the portal system, which flows into the liver. This means that, depending on the position within the rectum, only some of the drug absorbed from the rectum will be subject to the first pass effect. Bioavailability therefore may be less than 100%, but may be better than that obtained from other parts of the GIT.

The amount of fluid present in the rectum is small, estimated at approximately 3 mL of mucus. This affects the rate of dissolution of the drug released from the suppository. However, there is also muscular movement which spreads the drug over a large area and promotes absorption.

The advantages and disadvantages of this route of administration are as follows.

Advantages

- Can be used when the oral route is unsuitable, e.g. severe vomiting, unconscious patient, with uncooperative patients, such as children, the elderly or those with mental impairment, and patients with dysphagia

- Useful when the drug causes GIT irritation
- Can be used for local action.

Disadvantages

- Absorption can be irregular and unpredictable, giving rise to a variable effect
- Less convenient than the oral route
- There is low patient acceptability of this route in the UK. A wider acceptance is found in other parts of the world.

The vaginal route

For administration by this route, drugs may be formulated as pessaries, tablets, capsules, solutions, sprays, creams, ointments and foams, which are inserted into the vagina. Most often this route is used for a local effect. However, drugs absorbed from the vagina are not subject to the first pass effect and can give systemic bioavailability better than with the oral route.

The inhalation route

Drugs are administered usually by inhalation through the nose or mouth to produce either local or systemic effects. This route is used predominantly for local administration to treat respiratory conditions, such as asthma. For this, drugs are delivered directly to the site of action, i.e. the lungs. A variety of dosage forms are used, from simple inhalations consisting of volatile ingredients, such as menthol, to sophisticated inhaler devices (see Ch. 14). A major benefit of the inhaled route is that the drug dose required to produce the desired effect is much smaller than for the oral route, with a consequent reduction in side-effects. Because of the high blood flow to the lungs and their large surface area, drug absorption by this route is extremely rapid and can be used to give systemic action.

The nasal route

The nasal cavity has been traditionally used for producing local effects using solutions as drops or sprays. More recently, it has been used for systemic action because of its good vascular supply, which avoids first pass metabolism (e.g. calcitonin), although it does have some local enzymic activity.

The topical route

In the topical route, the skin is used as the site of administration. This route is most commonly used for local effects using liquid and powder dosage forms, in addition to the traditional ointments, creams and pastes (see Ch. 8). The skin has a natural barrier function, but specialized dosage forms have been developed which, when applied to the skin, allow the drug to pass through and produce a systemic effect. This avoids first pass effects and can produce close to zero-order kinetics over prolonged time intervals. (A more detailed discussion of this route of administration can be found in Ch. 8.)

The parenteral route

This is the term used to describe drug administration by injection. Within this general term, there is a variety of different routes. The main ones are:

- *Intravenous route*, where drugs are injected directly into the systemic circulation. This produces a very fast onset of action
- *Subcutaneous route*, where drugs are injected into the subcutaneous layer of the skin. This is the easiest and least painful type of injection to administer
- *Intramuscular route*, where drugs are injected into muscle layers. This method can be used to produce a fairly fast onset of action when the drug is formulated as an aqueous solution. A slower and more prolonged action will occur when the drug is presented as a suspension or in an oily vehicle.

These and other specialized types of injection are discussed more fully in Chapter 12.

Dosage forms

Drugs are presented in a wide variety of dosage forms. How a drug is formulated is dependent on a variety of factors, and the same drugs may be presented in several different dosage forms. It is important for pharmacists to appreciate the different properties of the varying dosage forms, in order that the most appropriate or most acceptable formulation is given to the patient. This section gives brief information on the different types of dosage forms. Additional, more detailed, information is found in the chapters dealing with specific formulations.

Aerosols

These consist of pressurized packs which contain the drug in solution or suspension and a suitable propellant. They are most commonly used for their local effect in the treatment of asthma. These devices are fitted with a metering valve, which allows a known dose of drug to be delivered each time the device is fired. Some aerosols are for topical use, particularly in the treatment of muscle sprains and injuries. These may contain substances, such as non-steroidal anti-inflammatory drugs or counter-irritants.

Applications

This is the name given to solutions, suspensions or emulsions which are for topical use. They contain substances such as ascaricides or antiseptics.

Capsules

These are solid dosage forms, generally for oral use. Some drugs formulated as capsules are intended to be inhaled. It is therefore important to inform the patient on their appropriate use. For both types of capsule, the drug is contained in a gelatin shell, usually as a powder or a liquid. Modified-release preparations are available where the drug is presented in the gelatin container, as small pellets with different coatings.

Collodions

These are liquid preparations for external use. The liquid is painted on the skin, where it forms a flexible film. They contain substances such as salicylic acid, which is useful in the treatment of corns.

Creams

These are semi-solid emulsions for external use. Because of the water content they are susceptible to microbial contamination and either include a preservative or are given a short shelf-life. Creams are easier to apply and are less greasy than ointments, so patients often prefer them.

Dusting powders

These are finely divided powders for external use. Their main uses are as lubricants, to prevent friction between skin surfaces and for disinfection and antisepsis in minor wounds.

Ear drops

These are used topically to treat a variety of ear problems. The drug, or mixture of drugs, is presented as a solution or suspension in a suitable vehicle such as water, glycerol, propylene glycol or alcohol. The drops are inserted into the ear, using a dropper. Some vehicles, such as alcohol, may cause a degree of stinging when applied to the ear. It is important to ensure that the patient is aware of this and is assured that it is a normal sensation. If patients find the degree of stinging unacceptable, they may have to be given ear drops with an aqueous vehicle. Oils, such as almond or olive, are often

recommended for the alleviation of impacted earwax. It is usually suggested that such oils should be warmed before being dropped into the ear. This can be done by holding the container between the hands and rubbing it for a few seconds.

Elixirs

An elixir is a solution of one or more drugs for oral use. The vehicle generally contains a high proportion of sucrose or, increasingly nowadays, a 'sugar-free' vehicle such as sorbitol solution, which is less likely to cause dental caries. The therapeutic action of drugs presented as elixirs varies widely and includes antihistamines, antibiotics and decongestants.

Emulsions

These are mixtures of two immiscible liquids, usually oil and water. When the term 'emulsion' is used, this refers to a preparation for oral use.

Enemas

An enema is an oily or aqueous solution which is administered rectally. A number of drugs are formulated as enemas and are used to treat conditions such as constipation or ulcerative colitis. They are also used in X-ray examination of the lower bowel and for systemic effects, such as the use of diazepam in status epilepticus and febrile convulsions.

Eye drops and eye ointments

These are sterile preparations used to administer drugs to the eye.

Gargles

Gargles are aqueous solutions used to treat infections of the throat. They are often presented in a concentrated form with instructions to the patient for dilution. Gargles should not be swallowed, but held in the throat while exhaling through the liquid. After a suitable time period, usually a minute or so, the patient should spit out the gargle.

Gels

Gels are semi-solid dosage forms for topical or other local use. They are usually transparent or translucent and have a variety of uses. Spermicides and lubricants are often presented in a gel form. Many patients prefer this formulation because it is non-greasy.

The term 'gel' is also used to describe colloidal suspensions of drugs such as aluminium and magnesium hydroxides.

Granules

This term is used to describe a drug which is presented in small irregularly-shaped particles. Granules may be packed in individual sachets, containing a unit dose of medicament, or may be provided in a bulk format, where the dose is measured using a 5-mL spoon. Some laxatives are among the drugs currently presented as granules.

Implants

This term refers to solid dosage forms, which are inserted under the skin by a small surgical incision. They are most commonly used for hormone replacement therapy or as a contraceptive. Release of the drug from implants is generally slow and long-term therapy is achieved. In the case of the contraceptive implant, the effect continues for up to 3 years. A testosterone implant, used in the treatment of male hypogonadism, will maintain adequate hormone levels in the patient for 4–5 months. Implants must be sterile.

Inhalations

These are preparations which contain volatile medicaments, which may have a beneficial effect in upper respiratory tract disorders such as nasal congestion. Some inhalations contain substances that are volatile at room temperature and the patient can obtain a degree of relief by adding a few drops to a handkerchief or a pillowcase and breathing in the vapour. Other inhalations are added to hot water and the impregnated steam is then inhaled. Many users of the latter type of inhalation use boiling water. Pharmacists should advise against this, as the steam produced is too hot and can damage the delicate mucous membranes of the upper respiratory tract. Overuse of this type of preparation should also be avoided, as it may cause a chronic condition to develop. The use of these strong aromatic decongestants is not advised in the BNF in children under 3 months, owing to the risk of apnoea.

Injections

These are used parenterally and are sterile (see Ch. 12).

Irrigations

These are sterile solutions most commonly used in the treatment of infected bladders. Sterile solutions of sodium chloride 0.9% (physiological saline) are used to treat a wide range of common urinary tract pathogens. Antifungal drugs, such as amphotericin and locally acting cytotoxics, e.g. doxorubicin and mitomycin, are introduced into the bladder as irrigations, to treat mycotic infections and bladder tumours, respectively.

Linctuses

A linctus is a viscous liquid for oral use, the majority being for the relief of cough. The viscous nature of the preparation coats the throat and helps to alleviate the irritation which is causing the problem. Previously, many linctuses contained a high level of sucrose; however, many have been reformulated as 'sugar-free' products, to reduce the risk of dental caries. Because the viscous nature of linctuses is beneficial, they should not be diluted prior to administration.

Liniments

These are liquids for external use. They are used to alleviate the discomfort of muscle strains and injuries. Because of the rubefacient nature of some of the ingredients, some sportsmen will use them prior to starting a sporting activity, in an attempt to avoid any muscle damage. Examples of active ingredients found in liniments are turpentine oil and methyl salicylate. The BNF states that the evidence around topical rubefacients does not support their use in acute or chronic musculoskeletal pain.

Lotions

These are liquids for external use and may be solutions, suspensions or emulsions. They have a variety of uses, which include antiseptic, parasiticidal and soothing. Care should be taken when recommending lotions for the treatment of head lice. Those which have an alcohol base should be avoided in asthmatics and young children, as the alcoholic fumes may cause breathing difficulties. Aqueous-based products should be advised.

Lozenges

These are large tablets designed to be sucked and remain in the mouth for up to 15 min. They do not contain a disintegrant and the active ingredient is normally incorporated into a sugar base, such as sucrose or glucose. The main use of lozenges is in the treatment of mouth and throat infections.

Mixtures

This is a generic term used for many liquid preparations for oral use.

Mouthwashes

These are similar in formulation to gargles, but are used specifically to treat conditions of the mouth. The active ingredients are usually antiseptics or bactericidal agents.

Nasal drops and sprays

These are isotonic solutions used to treat conditions of the nose. Locally acting decongestants are commonly presented as nose drops. The container includes a dropper device to allow the patient to deliver the appropriate dose into the affected nostril(s). Overuse of nose drops is common as patients find it difficult to judge the number of drops being delivered. Other preparations for both local and systemic use are presented as sprays (metered or pump).

Ointments

Ointments are semi-solids for topical use.

Paints

Paints are solutions for application to the skin. Those used on the skin are often formulated with a volatile vehicle. This evaporates on application and leaves a film of active ingredient on the skin surface.

Pastes

These are semi-solids for external use. They differ from creams and ointments in that they contain a high proportion of fine powder, such as starch. This makes them very stiff and means they do not spread readily over the skin's surface. Corrosive drugs, such as dithranol are often formulated as pastes, so that paste applied to the psoriatic lesion will not spread onto healthy skin and cause irritation.

Pastilles

Pastilles are for oral use and, like lozenges, are designed to be sucked. They contain locally acting antiseptics, astringents or anaesthetics and are used to treat, or give symptomatic relief from, conditions affecting the mouth and throat. They have a jelly-like consistency produced by their basis of gelatin or acacia.

Pessaries

Pessaries are solid dosage forms for insertion into the vagina. They are used for both local and systemic action.

Pills

Pills are a moulded oral dosage form, which has been superseded by tablets and capsules. The term is still used by the general public, incorrectly, to describe any solid oral dose form.

Powders (oral)

These occur as both bulk and divided powders. Bulk powders usually contain non-potent active ingredients, such as antacids. The dose is measured using a 5-mL spoon.

Individual powders are used for more potent drugs, where accuracy of dosage is more important. An individual dose is packaged separately, either in a sheet of paper or in a sachet.

Suppositories

These are solid dosage forms for insertion into the rectum. They are used for both local and systemic actions.

Suspensions

Suspensions are liquid dose forms where the active ingredient is insoluble. Suspensions are available for both oral and external use.

Syrups

These are concentrated aqueous solutions of sugars such as sucrose. The term 'syrup' is frequently, but incorrectly, applied to certain sweetened liquids intended for oral use. The term 'syrup' should nowadays only be used to refer to flavouring vehicles. Sucrose is being replaced by sorbitol as the sweetening agent in many preparations, to give 'sugar-free' syrups to reduce the risk of dental caries.

Tablets

This is the term used to describe compressed solid dosage forms generally intended for oral use, although some pessaries are tablets for vaginal use. As well as the standard tablet made by compression, there are many different types of tablet designed for specific uses, e.g. dispersible, gastro-resistant (enteric coated), modified release or buccal.

Transdermal delivery systems

This term is used to describe the adhesive patches which, when applied to the skin, deliver a controlled dose of drug over a specified time period to produce a systemic effect.

Administration of oral liquid medicines

Oral liquid medicines should come supplied with a standard size 5-mL medicine spoon, which has to conform to certain specifications. Household teaspoons should never be used to measure medicines, as they come in a variety of sizes, holding varying volumes of liquids. In some cases, it may be more appropriate to supply an oral syringe, for example if the volume of liquid to be administered is less than 5 mL, or if the patient is unable to take medicine from a spoon.

Key points

- The route can be chosen to give local or systemic effects, fast or slow onset, and is influenced by biopharmacy and pharmacokinetics
- The oral route is the most commonly used route
- Gastric emptying, stability and other materials present in the GIT may limit availability of the drug from the oral route

- Sublingual absorption gives a short, fast-onset activity
- Buccal absorption takes place between the gum and lip
- Buccal routes of administration can be used with unconscious patients and to avoid first pass metabolism
- Rectal absorption partially avoids first pass metabolism
- Rectal administration is useful for nil-by-mouth patients and in cases of gastric irritation. However, it is poorly accepted in the UK
- Vaginal administration can give systemic effects avoiding first pass metabolism
- Inhalation requires a much lower dose than the oral route, with a rapid onset
- Administration to the skin may be used for both local and systemic effects
- Injections can give the fastest onset of action, but prolonged action is also possible using oily intramuscular injections
- A wide range of different dosage forms, which have different properties and uses, has been devised
- The same drug may usefully be used in different formulations to assist different types of patients

Index

Note: Page numbers followed by "f" indicate figures, "t" indicate tables, and "b" indicate boxes.

Index

160

Index